The Irritable Bowel Syndrome (I.B.S.) & Gastrointestinal Solutions Handbook

by

Chet Cunningham

United Research Publishers

Published by United Research Publishers

Copyright © 2002, 1995 by Chet Cunningham

ISBN 0-961492-9-X

Library of Congress Control Number 95-60171

Printed and bound in the United States of America

This book is not intended to be a substitute for medical advice or treatment. Self-diagnosis can be dangerous. If you have a serious health problem, see your doctor or health care provider promptly.

Book design by The Final Draft, Encinitas, CA

Cover design by The Art Department, Encinitas, CA

Order additional copies of *The Irritable Bowel Syndrome (IBS) & Gastrointestinal Solutions Handbook* from:

> United Research Publishers
> P.O. Box 232344
> Encinitas CA 92023-2344

or on the Web at:

> www.unitedresearchpubs.com

Full 90-day money back guarantee if not satisfied.

CONTENTS

INTRODUCTION

YOU'RE FEELING TERRIBLE. Your stomach is churning. You're afraid you might throw up. Yesterday you had such a case of constipation that you wanted to scream. Last week it was cramps and spasms in your gut and no matter what you ate or didn't eat the ugly, sick feeling just wouldn't go away.

You have some of the classic symptoms of Irritable Bowel Syndrome often called I.B.S. These are fancy words that mean your gut hurts, you can't make it stop and sometimes you want to throw things and hit people.

More than 80 million Americans suffer from I.B.S. or some other chronic digestive problem. Many have more than one of the umbrella of aches, pains and conditions that are grouped together and called I.B.S. The big problem is that most people don't understand their medical condition, don't know how it came about and, most importantly, don't have the slightest idea what to do about it.

More women than men get I.B.S. We're not sure why. It might be that more women complain about it and go see doctors, while the men try to macho it out.

After the common cold, I.B.S. and digestive tract complaints cause the most visits to doctor offices. Symptoms can come and go, perhaps for months before many people seek medical help.

Unfortunately problems with the digestive system upset a person's whole way of life. They can involve meals, family outings, social events, business and sports activities. If you need to run to the bathroom every hour, you won't be much good to your team whether it's a business, sports or social group.

Many times the pleasures of eating a good meal are ruined because you worry about what a certain food is going to do to your bowels. If you eat something that's disagreed with you before, you can bet that it will do so again.

The fact is clear that I.B.S. is a serious problem. No, it's not a disease, it's a condition. A condition that can drive you crazy, and usually one that can last for years and years. Some aspects of I.B.S. probably crept up on you so gradually you didn't realize it. Most of the uglier symptoms of it can be controlled, reduced in severity and made fit to live with.

Yes, stress and pressure can make your I.B.S. worse. But then that same stress can make a person without I.B.S. suddenly feel sick to his or her stomach, or rush to the bathroom with a sudden case of diarrhea. Yes, we know that the mind affects the body, it's called psychosomatic, and it's terribly real. But I.B.S. is not the result of conditions that are all in your mind.

You have actual, undeniably severe physical ailments

that can and should be treated. That's part of what we're going to be talking about in this book, so just hang on and we'll get there, or skip to that section in the Contents Page that most nearly reflects your grungy feeling to date and study it carefully.

I.B.S., digestion problems and trouble with your colon can strike anyone in any income or educational level, regardless of your place of birth, religious, political, racial background, or even your favorite baseball team. I.B.S. is the most democratic of conditions.

More than half of the victims of I.B.S. are between the ages of twenty-four and forty-six, and sixty percent of those cases are women.

Stomach pains, cramps, passing air, burping, heartburn, spasms, queasiness, flip-flopping between constipation and diarrhea, acid rising in your throat, tender abdomen, sharp belly pains, vomiting, excessive tiredness and unexplained backache, are all conditions that most doctors group under the I.B.S. label.

We'll be covering each of these conditions in detail and as we move along, show what you may be able to do yourself to help reduce the severity of the conditions or perhaps eliminate them all together.

The problems with I.B.S. can range anywhere from a mild upset to something so serious that hospitalization is needed and often a pain killing drug such as morphine must be prescribed to give the patient relief.

In many cases a condition might easily be misdiagnosed as being one problem, but the doctor checks and finds absolutely nothing wrong in that area. This should not happen. The I.B.S. conditions should be viewed as a part of the whole and treated as a series of conditions over a time span, not as one problem.

The first step in any such treatment must be to do the standard tests to make sure there is no complicated disease of the digestive tract that's causing the problems. When those diseases are eliminated, work can start to bring the I.B.S. problems under control.

At times a patient will go from doctor to doctor with the problem. Or HMOs or large organizations will pass a patient around with a lot of head wagging that it "isn't anything in my specialty." Sometimes the final doctor has to say that he's just not sure what the problem is and that the patient is going to have to learn to live with it.

Don't you believe them. Find a doctor who knows about the wily and complicated nature of I.B.S. and who understands the frustrations of its treatments for the doctor as well as for the patient. Then you'll have a chance to get some kind of satisfaction.

When the final push comes to shove, it may be that you are the best one to treat yourself, since you know intimately and with full understanding just how your symptoms are torturing you. We hope to help you to help yourself with this book of answers, even if no one else can.

In this book you'll learn that sometimes your worrying about I.B.S. can be as bad as the condition itself. You'll be told in plain terms that no one has ever died of I.B.S. Also there is no real indications that I.B.S. leads to any serious diseases of the bowel such as cancer or Crohn's disease. One more caution you'll hear about is that a problem shared is a problem cut in half. So share your I.B.S. condition with your friends and your doctor. Some of your best friends may have the same problems that you do.

Perhaps you have a more dangerous problem with your gastrointestinal tract, such as an ulcer and a bad gallbladder. The treatment for one can often upset the other one. There is nothing simple about the gastro system and its intricate orchestration of dozens of different jobs to give you a smooth operating digestive experience.

Any idea what the best selling drug in the world is? For the past several years it has been a race between two drugs, both of them help control the stomach acid problem. The leader is Zantac with sales of over 2 BILLION DOLLARS a year. Close behind is the runner up, Tagamet, now at 1.2 BILLION DOLLARS in sales a year.

Why do they sell so much of these drugs? Because up to 80 million people in the U. S. alone are regular customers who take the drugs to try to kill their acid stomachs.

So, be of good cheer. We're going to touch on your exact problem, and we hope offer some solid, practical ways to make you feel better and to beat the long term effects of your I.B.S.

So you'll have a solid base to know what we're talking about, we'll be doing a little bit of Health 102, some instructional details, basic training about what your gastrointestinal tract is, exactly what elements make it up, and where they are all situated in your body.

Once we have that foundation, we'll move on to show you in layman's terms just how your gastrointestinal tract works. This trip will take us down the route from your mouth to your esophagus into your stomach and all the way through to the end of the line at the anus.

On that trip you'll find out what goes on in your stomach, in your small and large intestines, and something of the problems that can come up. With the problems will be some treatments.

Then we want to show you a list of two dozen complaints that a lot of people have. You can check along and see how you fit in with this ultra detailed list of almost every problem you can have or feel in your digestive system.

After that, we take a close look at this problem called Irritable Bowel Syndrome. As we said before, it's a term that is used as a catchall for at least ten or twelve common complaints by patients about their bowels, stomach and their digestive system as a whole.

Some people say that they can stop your stomach and bowel distress in seven days by controlling what you eat. This might be true in a few cases where not much is wrong, but most I.B.S. patients need a lot more help than to just stop eating apple peelings or milk or wheat products.

In this section of the book we'll try to cover all of the symptoms that I.B.S. patients complain about. We'll go into detail about gas and bloating, nausea and vomiting, heartburn, gut pain on empty, gut pain on over full, diarrhea, constipation, anal problems, antacids and Giardia parasites, tender abdomen, sharp belly pain, excessive tiredness and unexplained backache.

Diet has been mentioned as one component of the I.B.S. situation. Whole books have been written around the idea that your diet is the total controlling factor in all of your gut problems.

We don't go that far, but we will point out that there are certain conditions of the human gut that can be helped by a different diet. However, there are many other elements involving your digestive tract that have nothing to do with food.

The problem becomes even more complex when we show you that some food will throw one person into spasms, diarrhea and terrible pain, while the same food and conditions with someone else will have no affect at all.

Most authorities today agree that there are seven deadly sins that many people commit to hurt their own gut. These become trigger situations that can make many people's I.B.S much better or much worse depending how they treat these seven situations and habits. At the end of this section we show how too much fat in the diet is unhealthy for the I.B.S. patient as for anyone else. A chart of some twenty pages will be in an appendix at the end of the book to show you just how many fat grams are lurking in most of our food today.

Later in the book we'll talk about the diseases of the digestive tract. These are recognized and treatable diseases, not like the I.B.S. conditions that affect your digestive system. Here we detail the problems with ulcers, gall bladder, colitis, diverticulosis, esophagus, hiatus hernia, worms, malabsorption, hemorrhoids, appendicitis, cancer of the digestive tract, food poisoning and food allergies.

These are diseases that require the attention of a doctor and since they have a solid cause, are often easier to treat than the I.B.S. problems, which can be individualistic, spasmodic and infuriatingly diverse, hidden and mystifying even to gastroenterology specialists.

The last section of the book shows some of the non-traditional helps and ideas that might be of some aid in your fight against I.B.S. and your other gut problems.

These include: homeopathy helps, relaxation ideas, the aging G.I. tract, traveling and your gut, hypnotherapy, aromatherapy, herbal helps and even acupuncture.

This is an answer book, designed to give you some aid and comfort and some answers to some of your gastro-intestinal problems. Don't worry, this isn't a move to cut out your doctor. But the fact remains that many of the I.B.S. symptoms are of a type that often can be reduced and even eliminated by yourself taking into consideration many of the suggestions that will be made in this book.

Yes, you should see your doctor, but many doctors don't have the time, or patience to "fool around" with a patient who has an upset stomach now and then and some occasional diarrhea. We want you to know all you can about how you can help yourself to solve or reduce the severity of as many of your gut conditions as you can before you go see your doctor.

So, you're off on your adventure down the self-help trail to a better digestive system. We hope that this book can help, and that you'll be living a more comfortable and productive life down the road.

Read on!

1
WHAT'S A GASTRO-INTESTINAL TRACT?

FIRST LET'S SHORTEN that long medically sounding word to G.I. tract. Sometimes it might be just "gastro," but you'll know what we mean. Now for hundreds of years the people who go around making people well have called the G.I. tract a long tube, one with a few bulges and pockets and twists and turns that runs for a little over twenty-seven feet from your throat to your anus.

Nothing wrong with the word "anus," a good, solid Latin word from the 15th century meaning "the posterior opening of the alimentary canal."

STARTING AT THE TOP: THE ESOPHAGUS

With that out of the way, we move downward. We can start at the mouth and the throat, but you know about them. Then we come to the esophagus. This is really where the G.I. tract begins. The esophagus is not much more than a sixteen inch long tube that's about an inch wide.

When you start to swallow, a valve closes off your air

tube to your lungs and larynx so the food goes down your esophagus. It has a tough mucus-membrane lining much like the inside of your mouth. This mucus coats the food as it descends helping it pass and protecting your esophagus from abrasive foods, bits of bone, hard food or sharp seeds.

You swallow something and the muscles in your esophagus grab the food and push it toward the stomach. No, just swallowing doesn't get that food into your stomach, the muscles in your esophagus do that automatically. This is called peristaltic contractions and they move the food and liquids along even if you are lying down or standing on your head.

Fluids and chewed up foods move down your esophagus in six or seven seconds. On the other hand dry food can take up to fifteen minutes. Maybe the water you drink after dry foods slides right past it.

When that bite of food we were talking about is pushed down to the end of the tube it comes to a one way trap door called a sphincter that opens, letting the food through and then snaps closed so nothing below it can get back up your esophagus. That's the way it's supposed to work, but we'll show you later what happens when something goes wrong with that trap door.

The esophagus is literally a corridor, a highway, for food and liquids. It doesn't do anything else, does not secrete or absorb, or store food or digest anything. Into the mouth, over the tongue, watch out, esophagus, here it comes!

NEXT, THE STOMACH

Once past the long tube, the food hits the stomach. Your stomach is a muscular bag that begins just below the notch in your breastbone, left of center, where it connects with the esophagus and it ends where it empties into the small intestine.

Your stomach is more than a storage warehouse. It has four vital functions:

1. It does store food and liquids.
2. It secretes acids to aid digestion.
3. It mixes and churns the food and acids.
4. It contains stomach acid that kills most of the bacteria that were swallowed with the food and liquids.

Most experts agree that storage is the most important function of the stomach. It can hold from one to one and a half quarts. The stomach can stretch or shrink in size depending on the amount of food that is taken in. An anorexia nervosa victim might have a shrunken stomach that would hold less than one cup of fluid and food. Some large individuals have been tested to show that they have stomachs that will hold six quarts.

Some individuals have their stomachs removed due to illness. They can survive, but must eat and drink small amounts of food and liquids since there's no storage area.

The stomach secretes a highly concentrated form of

hydrochloric acid. True. Scientists still wonder how a living organism can do such a thing. This acid activates the stomach to produce pepsin, its major digestive enzyme. The acid and the pepsin both attack the proteins to break them down.

How do you survive the hydrochloric acid in your belly? There's a mucus shield in the stomach and evidently this acts as a barrier between the acid and the stomach wall tissue so no harm is done, and only the protein feels the power of the acid.

Some experts say that the stomach has a protective system called cytoprotection. The gurus say that in the mucus are prostaglandins. These are powerful chemical messengers which can either start or stop cellular activity. Evidently they are in the thick mucus stomach lining and give a chemical shield that protects the stomach's walls, yet lets the hydrochloric acid chew up everything else.

Our experts also say that the prostaglandins also help your stomach lining repair itself. Each meal wears out part of your stomach's mucus lining and the prostaglandins help it start generating new cells six to eight hours after every meal.

Now the stomach walls work on the food by squeezing it and mixing it with the acid and gastric juices and enzymes. Usually about two hours after a meal, the food has been reduced to a liquid state and moved toward the small intestine.

Exceptions. High protein foods, such as meat, can take up to four hours to move through the stomach. A high fat meal can mean up to six hours of stomach work before it's ready to move on. It simply takes the stomach that much longer to break down the more complicated fat and protein materials into a liquid for processing downstream.

Some interesting sidelights. Your stomach is stuffed with about two gallons of food and liquids over the course of a day. That's over forty tons of food and drink in an average lifetime. Food can take from twenty-four hours all the way up to ninety-eight hours (that's four days!), to travel through your digestive tract. The saliva glands in your mouth secrete a little over a quart of fluid a day. That means you'll be swallowing from 2,300 to 2,400 times a day just to move the saliva.

We mentioned that the stomach acids can kill bacteria. True. But it doesn't take care of all of them. With a massive number of bacteria, such as is in salmonella food poisoning, the stomach can't kill all of them, and you get sick. Some other potent disease germs such as those for cholera, can pass through the stomach unscathed.

Tapeworm and hookworms are undisturbed by the stomach acids and for the most part viruses and parasites are less affected by the stomach fighters.

THE SMALL INTESTINE

Next in the chain of operation comes the small intestine. The small intestine is vital to your health, safety and welfare. Without it you couldn't live. They can cut out your stomach, remove most of your large intestine, and you'll live and can thrive. But without your small intestine, none of the food you eat would be absorbed so the body could use it.

The whole process works this way. The food mixture enters the small intestine, in the first section known as the duodenum. Here it is flooded with juices from the pancreas that neutralizes the acid mixture to protect the small intestine and so it can then work on the food mixture.

Now the pancreas takes over again and secretes exactly the correct enzymes and in the right amounts and at the right times to break down the kind and type of food that you've eaten. A computer couldn't do it better.

Enzymes? New word? That is a chemical that makes things happen without getting involved itself. Like a catalyst. Every second we live, millions of chemical reactions are taking place inside our bodies. We repair tissue, build new tissue, assemble and break down molecules and all sorts of things.

The enzymes help these changes take place without the violent reactions you'd get in a test tube if the same chemicals were allowed to work uncontrolled.

Once the enzymes have done their job on that food

mixture, the carbohydrates and proteins are ready to be used by your body. The fats that you've eaten need more work and that comes when the liver secretes bile to dissolve those fats. Bile is made by the liver and stored in your gallbladder.

Food in your small intestine stimulates the gallbladder which dumps the right amount of bile into the intestine to use on the fats.

The small intestine is not just twenty-one feet of smooth tubing. Your small intestine is a highly complex system. It is lined with thousands of velvet-like accordion folds. Each one of these folds has millions of extremely small threads coming out from them called villi. The surface of a shag rug or a fine towel would be a good comparison.

Each of these tiny thread villi is in turn covered with thousands of even smaller thread-like projections called microvilli, or smaller villi. These tiny threads each contain a surging supply of blood.

Experts have estimated that a square inch of the small intestine's lining holds 20,000 villi and over 10 billion microvilli. This means that the active surface of the small intestine is multiplied tremendously and makes it a highly efficient manufacturing device. Man-made machines don't even come into the same playing field of complexity with the small intestine.

The job of these tiny threads is to utilize 95 percent of the nutrients in the food and liquids that you take in daily. They do it by what the medical world calls absorption.

Sugars, amino acids and electrolytes are absorbed easily by the tiny microvilli swaying in the watery tide influx of the food slurry. They pass through the villi and into your bloodstream.

Fats are tougher. They must be absorbed by lymph vessels in the walls of the small intestine. The fats pass through the lymph vessels into the blood and are moved to the liver.

The liver works on all of the nutrients it gets from the blood and changes them into forms your body can use as fuel. That's one reason your liver is so vital to your good health.

By the time the food stuff mixture has worked its way past those billions of microvilli and moved to the far end of the small intestine, about ninety-five percent of it has been absorbed. When your system works correctly, all of the food value has been wrung out of that meal, and the indigestible parts that are left are passed on into the large intestine.

YOUR COLON OR LARGE INTESTINE

Your colon is the final section of your G.I. tract. It stretches five feet and accepts the food mixture from your small intestine where it passes through a one way valve. Near this entry way is the appendix.

This small organ has no known function, but is made up of lots of lymph tissue and some experts say it really does have a purpose, we just don't know what it is yet. The appendix can become infected and enlarge and without treatment can burst and release dangerous fluids into your body that can be fatal.

In the past a healthy appendix was often removed when doctors were operating in that area, to "prevent any future trouble." Now this isn't done as much as the experts ponder the purpose of the appendix.

When the end of this food mixture reaches your large intestine, most of the nutrients have already been absorbed from it. The colon does not digest, so no digestive juices are secreted. It does produce mucus to help lubricate the passage of the material.

The large intestine does absorb water from the mixture. Your body floods your food intake with water, digestive juices and saliva. A normal adult has about two and a half gallons of fluid pass into the colon every day.

Some eighty percent of this fluid is soaked up and absorbed by the colon daily, putting it back into your system. Remember your blood is ninety percent water and your whole body is seventy percent water. It's always in need of more water.

The residue in your colon is contracting. There are some useful bacteria in your colon on a normal basis. Some remove vitamin K from the food remains and send it into your bloodstream. Other bacteria can synthesize Vitamin B but not in large amounts.

Passing through your colon, your waste products keep losing water and reduce in size. Some sixty percent of the volume is still water along with fruit skins, seeds, fiber, sloughed off cells and old linings of your G.I. tract.

The fiber you eat helps to keep your colon full and it works most efficiently that way. The fiber also helps to soften your stool so it can move easier along the tube.

The same action of the small intestine that moves the material along, peristalsis, works in the colon as well. However here it is not continuous, but gets into motion whenever needed to move waste products along the five foot length of the colon.

When the stool enters the foot long rectum area, the walls of the usually empty store room stretch. This triggers your urge to have a bowel movement.

The anus is the far end of the G.I. tract. It is another sphincter and normally is tightly closed most of the time. You relax it when you need to have a movement.

TWO MORE IMPORTANT ORGANS OF THE G.I. TRACT

THE GALLBLADDER

We mentioned briefly how the gallbladder contributes to digestion. A few more details.

The gallbladder is located just below your right ribs and is a sack about the size of an adult thumb. It stores and concentrates bile, a green fluid that is produced by the liver.

When food enters the first section of the small intestine from the stomach, it triggers the gallbladder to contract. This pushes bile into the intestine where it helps digest fats.

This is one of the organs that we can live without. If there is no gallbladder, the bile from the liver will seep into the small intestine twenty-four hours a day. So digestion would continue at a normal pace. When the bile has done its job in the first sections of the small intestine, most of it is absorbed in the lower part of the intestine and reprocessed. Your body recycles. A small part of the bile continues on to the colon where it gives the stool the brown coloration.

THE PANCREAS

This long gland lays in the curve of the first part of the small intestine and tails away to the left. The pancreas makes insulin and it also produces digestive juices. Between one and four quarts of these juices are secreted into the intestine every day. They help and aid in digestion.

People can live without a pancreas, but that generates several problems. It can be marked as one of the non-essential organs for continued life.

So, that wraps up the educational section about what your G.I. tract is and what it does. Now we move on to the material that is going to help you kill off or severely damage around the head and shoulders the Irritable Bowel Syndrome or other G.I. tract problems that have been plaguing you.

2
SOME GASTRO SYMPTOMS YOU MIGHT HAVE

BY NOW YOU SHOULD HAVE a sketchy idea of how your internal food to energy manufacturing plant works. As you know, sometimes the works get out of whack a little, something goes wrong and ... it hurts.

There are more than two dozen different ways that your G.I. tract can have problems, and many of these are conditions that you may be able to help yourself with a little self-care and some common sense.

Right up front let us emphasize that self-diagnosis is usually not a good idea. But if you're having some minor problem with constipation or flatulence, it could take some relatively simple changes in your life style or eating habits to solve the condition.

When you have pains or blood in your stool or other serious symptoms, be sure to see your doctor at once, because what you have could be a serious and even life-threatening disease.

When considering your digestive tract you might feel pressure, pain or spasms. You might suffer from constipation, diarrhea, bleeding, belching, flatulence and mild weight loss.

What we want to do here is to show some of the symptoms you might have and what they may mean. Just what to do about them we'll get to in later chapters.

If you have any type of dietary pains or problems and have not had a long talk with your doctor about them, you should take that course first. Tell your doctor exactly what your symptoms are and let him rule out any of the more serious G.I. tract diseases. If he or she can say you don't have one of the diseases of the digestive system, then you'll be relieved and ready to tackle these upsetting and disquieting digestive tract conditions. Chances are that you may be able to do a lot to take care of your feeling bad condition by yourself.

Here is a list of symptoms that patients have experienced. If you have any of these, you should talk to your doctor about them. Unfortunately many doctors are too busy these days to take the time and effort needed to solve or relieve many of the conditions of the digestive system that are not diseases and life threatening. If your doctor tells you it's all in your head or to eat more fiber, you probably should get a second opinion and try to see how you can help yourself.

SYMPTOMS OF G.I. TRACT DISTRESS

1. Do you sometimes taste undigested food as if you have regurgitated it without throwing up?

    If so it could mean that your sphincter valve in your esophagus isn't doing its job.

2. Do you have repeated feelings of pain in your right lower abdomen?

    It could be appendicitis, Crohn's disease, even ovarian cysts. Check with your doctor. If he says it's none of these three and it's Irritable Bowel Syndrome, be happy. Try some I.B.S. self help ideas.

3. Have your stools changed quite suddenly?

    If the stool is pencil thin, it might mean that there's a blockage in your colon that could be a tumor. See your doctor at once.

4. Have you lost fifteen or twenty pounds quite quickly without trying?

    Such a signal could mean a serious gastro disease. See your specialist at once.

5. Do you often find a sour taste in your mouth when you bend over or lie down?

    This means stomach acid has traveled up your esophagus into your mouth.

6. Do you sometimes experience severe itching around your anus?

   It might be hemorrhoids, or it could be pinworms. You can get them easily from small children. Talk to your doctor.

7. Do you have frequent and extended periods of loose stools, constipation alternating with diarrhea, or simply constipation?

   If this is a new problem, check with your doctor. If it's a long standing situation, check out the I.B.S. section.

8. Have you often awakened in the night coughing?

   This might mean acid from your stomach escaping into your esophagus is being pulled into your lungs when you are sleeping. Tell your doctor so he can rule out any heart or lung problems.

9. Do you see blood mixed in your stool rather than just streaked on the outside?

   If it doesn't come from your anal area it could be a tumor, polyp, or some inflammatory bowel disease. Consult with your doctor.

10. Are you over 40 and recently suffered from severe constipation?

    It could be a tumor blocking your colon. See your doctor. Sudden constipation might also come from travel, side effects of prescription drugs, or I.B.S.

11. Do you have heartburn under your breastbone at least once a week or so?

    Have your doctor check it out.

12. Do you suffer frequently from pain on both sides of your lower abdomen?

    Check with your doctor. If he says it's I.B.S. you can do a lot to relieve it yourself.

13. Do you experience chronic diarrhea and rectal bleeding?

    You should see your doctor at once. You could have ulcerated colitis, colon polyps, dysentery, bad hemorrhoids or some other inflammatory bowel disease.

14. Do some high acid foods and juices burn all the way down your esophagus?

    This could be that your esophagus is inflamed from acid reflux. Don't just avoid those foods. See your doctor first to rule out an infection of your esophagus.

15. Do you find blood on your toilet paper when you wipe?

    Blood there or on your stool usually means you have a fissure or hemorrhoids. It could be a serious problem like inflammatory bowel disease, so see your doctor at once.

16. Does it seem like you need to move your bowels many times a day, even after you've had one?

    It could be tenesmus which is caused by a partial blockage of the colon. Check with your doctor this week.

17. Do you have the annoying problem of belching frequently?

    It could be from swallowing air while eating, eating too fast, or just being up-tight. Not serious so try to relax. Don't swallow air when you eat or drink.

18. Do you pass air and embarrass yourself unmercifully?

    You might be able to control it with some dietary changes. See that chapter in the book.

19. Does your skin or the whites of your eyes have a yellowish tinge?

    If you do and have unusual itching, amber colored urine and light colored stools, you could have a liver or bile duct problem. See your doctor at once.

20. Do you feel full quickly after you start a meal?

    If this is recent, it could mean trouble of the doctoring kind. Make that appointment for a check.

21. If you have black or tarry bowel movements, it could mean a bleeding ulcer.

See your doctor as soon as possible.

22. Do you have any problem swallowing food or liquids?

    This could mean that your esophagus is obstructed in some way or not contracting the way it should. See your doctor.

23. Do you often have a tender abdomen?

    Check it out with your doctor, it could be a variety of problems, or not much at all.

24. Do sharp belly pains bother you?

    Talk it over with your doctor. I.B.S. helps may be the answer.

25. Do you have an unexplained backache that is chronic and just won't go away?

    Yes, it could be related to your gut more than your back. Check with your doctor.

3
A BRIEFING ON IRRITABLE BOWEL SYNDROME

THE NEXT SEVERAL CHAPTERS are going to go into detail about a variety of conditions that millions of people suffer from which doctors have grouped together into a phrase: Irritable Bowel Syndrome. This simply means a number of conditions that hurt people's gastrointestinal tracts.

Remember that key word "conditions." I.B.S. does not talk about or mean any "disease." We've said this before, but it must be plain and we want to be sure that you understand it.

What's the difference between a condition and a disease?

A sprained ankle is a condition, cancer is a disease. Belching is a condition, measles is a disease. A broken leg is a condition, AIDS is a disease.

A gastrointestinal condition might jump up and smite you because of any number of different reasons. The problem may hit you hard but that same cause may leave your brother, wife or friend totally unaffected.

The umbrella of a "syndrome" lets us group all of these conditions under one heading, so we can deal with them all or individually and keep them separated from the diseases of the digestive system that we'll talk about later.

I.B.S. is a highly complex problem for those who are affected and for their practitioners trying to treat it. It often shows up in the form of constipation, diarrhea, noisy stomach, heartburn, flatulence, gut pains, gas and bloating, nausea and vomiting, a tender abdomen and even unexplained back pains.

Many times one individual will have three or four of these problems all at once or over the course of a day.

Right up front let us say that there is no one "cure" for all of these conditions. Many times doctors will not agree on the cure or treatment for any one of the ailments. Today, with doctors as busy as they are, all too often the patient is hurried out the door with the admonition that they will "get better soon," or that "it's all in their head," or that "they will just have to live with it."

Some people say that I.B.S. is not life threatening so how bad can it be? It can be tremendously serious with the patient hospitalized and morphine drug treatments needed to control pain in some extreme cases.

Your doctor can do nothing for you unless you can tell him precisely how you feel, where it hurts, what happens, what foods you eat, if you're under any stress, and a few other details of your personal life that he or she needs to know.

Again, let us say that if you are a newcomer to I.B.S. problems, or an old hand going back perhaps decades, your first and best move is to go see your doctor. He or she can at least rule out the more deadly types of diseases of the bowel and the G.I. tract. If you know you don't have something, you're making progress and don't have to worry about that one.

A second step for you to take is to realize that you do have a medical problem, one that there is a solution to, and that it's not something that your spouse or your job or your boss has somehow caused and you haven't generated the whole thing in your mind. I.B.S. in any of its forms is not an inconvenience without a cure. Every one of the conditions can be reduced in severity, displaced entirely, or adjusted so you have a more normal life without the agonizing pain, social disasters, and embarrassment that many of the conditions can produce.

Part of the problem with beginners who have I.B.S. is that they do not believe that they have a medical problem. They see their situation as being brought on by some temporary cause, a bad lunch, work pressure, a fight with a spouse, a "low" feeling. They know that this upset will pass soon and they will be fine again. Probably just not true.

Your first step to getting well is to realize that you have a medical problem. The second step is to go to your doctor and talk it out, tell him or her exactly how you feel, where you hurt, all of your health-history. Then work with your physician on regaining your health.

A third step is to talk to your good friends about your problem. You will be surprised to find out how many people have some similar I.B.S. conditions. Those who know say that one of every four adults has some type of chronic or intermittent I.B.S. problem. True, the bowels are not usually considered a "nice" or proper topic of conversation, however that feeling is changing.

Now with talk radio delving into the most intimate sexual activity and personal health problems, the gastrointestinal area of health is much easier to talk about with friends. Give it a try, what do you have to lose?

One caution. Don't become obsessed with your condition. Don't worry it to death. Later we'll show that this worry can actually cause some physical problems, and it is sure to make others that you have even worse. Be concerned, but don't let the worry about it get you down.

Above all else, don't be concerned that a chronic sore esophagus is going to lead to cancer, or that a little blood in your stool means you have colon cancer. Get it checked out quickly by a doctor and put that worry behind you. Remember, nobody has ever died as a direct result of I.B.S.

With I.B.S. there is no "down the road" unpleasant cure for you to worry about. No chemotherapy, no machines to hook up to for cleansing your blood, no operations and painful recoveries. What you have to look forward to is relief and a complete healing in some situations, and in almost every aspect of I.B.S. there can be a downgrading of the condition making it a great deal easier to live with.

DIGGING A LITTLE DEEPER

Let's look at this I.B.S. monster in a little more depth. First, the term itself, "syndrome." Not a usual word. A syndrome is the combining form of two Greek words meaning running together. Generally it's a group of actions, emotions or events that form a pattern which are built up around a particular act.

So, all of the various conditions that irritate and plague the gut have been grouped together and called Irritable Bowel Syndrome.

No, you don't have them all at once. You may, however, have two or three at the same time, or in quick succession.

Next we need to mention the norm. What is normal in the G.I. tract? Normal is when all is going well and you don't even think about your digestive system. It's on automatic pilot and you don't have to think about or worry about what you eat or your social activities or your bowels in any way.

For example, normal bowel movements can range from once a day to once every four days. Some individuals' systems have been patterned so they automatically have two movements a day. There are people on record who have a normal bowel movement every thirty days. Amazing, but true. On the other hand, if you need to go to the bathroom every hour, and your whole life is centered around your bathroom at home and public restrooms and the toilets at work, you are in serious need of medical attention. This you don't have to live with.

Your bowels, like the rest of your body, are controlled by signals from your brain. Many of our bodily functions are automatically managed by the brain. We breathe and our hearts beat and we reach and move and walk, all without conscious direction.

We don't think: "Now, I want to move my hand over there. Brain, give me the signals to move it." We simply move the hand.

Your digestive system works much the same way. It's on automatic pilot, or a computer macro, and gets the job done. When something goes wrong, then we start getting signals from the brain that we need to take independent action. This might be a rush order to get to a toilet because the old colon is full and about to discharge.

While the brain gives the orders, you can over-ride those signals for a time, but the physical side is going to let you down from time to time.

Yes, your emotions have a part in all of this as well. You've heard about a witness in a big trial who suddenly gets sick to his stomach and has to leave the court in a rush so he can vomit. Sometimes extreme stress in a panic situation will cause a person to lose control of his or her bladder and wet pants result. Some rookie policemen and other cops who have never had to fire their guns or see a grisly murder scene, can suddenly have a case of uncontrollable diarrhea right there on the job and seriously embarrass themselves.

Emotions can and do affect our physical side. Our job is not to let them unduly affect our regular daily life.

Psychiatrists have patients who find that their emotions and the stress of tough situations cause all sorts of physical problems. Extended worry about a situation, a panic over a job loss, trouble with the boss at work, a difficult marital situation, all can be enough to trigger some sort of an I.B.S. upset.

It can be a serious problem with the mind setting off some I.B.S. condition, then we worry about it and make it worse than it was before. It can become a vicious circle. That's one way you can help yourself. Don't worry about your condition. Instead, go to your doctor, try to find the cause and work toward solving the problem, rather than making it worse by worrying.

WHAT ABOUT THE EFFECTS OF STRESS?

Yes, almost everyone agrees that stress is a highly important factor in many of our physical ills, I.B.S. included. Stress on the job, at home, with children, in your profession, even the stress of sociological problems, moral questions and religious conviction dilemmas, can all lead to an actual outbreak of some I.B.S. conditions.

Stress can be described as any situation an individual is in which tends to affect him negatively and changes his or her normal habit patterns, outlook and behavior.

We can see the evidence of stress in others. We might notice a fellow worker is drinking more than usual, that he or she is snapping at us, is irritable, hurried, tense, always on edge.

Some compare long term stress with short term hyper-activity when we get psyched up for a project, to win a game, to solve a problem or to win a race. We get a shot of adrenaline that gives us the spurt of energy to try to do the physical or mental job we've taken on.

Some experts say that this same type of "hyped" feeling when carried out on a long term basis from fear of losing a job, or anger at a boss or general frustration with someone, or even a growing unhappiness with a marriage, produces dangerous physical and psychological effects.

This tenseness over a period of time does the damage.

It can show up in any sort of way, many times not I.B.S. conditions but as a cough, in headaches, loss of appetite, and a host of other psychological and behavioral symptoms.

We're interested in those that could affect the I.B.S. conditions. Enough for us to say here that there can be such problems and causes of I.B.S. and that they should be something to check for as you talk with your doctor and work up your own self-help litany in your own fight against I.B.S.

Can you figure out if you have too much stress yourself? Try this handy self-analysis test. These are little habits that we normally wouldn't do and would find annoying in others. Take a look for some of these traits in yourself:

- ☐ Drumming fingers, tapping toes.
- ☐ Insomnia.
- ☐ Loss of appetite.
- ☐ Over eating.
- ☐ No sexual desire.
- ☐ Starting to smoke again.
- ☐ Drinking more than usual.
- ☐ Constantly licking your lips.
- ☐ Biting your fingernails.
- ☐ Staying in bed when awake.
- ☐ Loss of interest in work.
- ☐ Fast, shallow breathing.
- ☐ Jumping at normal sounds.
- ☐ Sweating with no cause.

- ☐ Dry, foul-tasting mouth.
- ☐ Holding your breath without knowing it.
- ☐ Pains in stomach, chest or neck for no reason.
- ☐ Hyper-sensitive to criticism.
- ☐ Can't concentrate.
- ☐ Worry over trivial happenings.
- ☐ Feeling inadequate, undervalued.
- ☐ Won't discuss your problems with others.
- ☐ A "fed up with it all" feeling.

Realizing that you are letting tense feelings get to you is the first step. Talk this over with your doctor as well. The medic probably knows that your being tense aggravates your I.B.S. problems.

Relieving long term stress is a field unto itself. If this is a big problem with you, there may be a need for psychological help first, and then see what that does for your I.B.S. conditions and take it from there.

Tension and stress are highly important in the battle with your I.B.S. Figure it out, realize you need help, make some effort today to get that help.

DO I REALLY HAVE I.B.S.?

We've said that everyone has some of the minor discomforts of I.B.S. from time to time. That includes you. So how do you figure out if you really have an I.B.S. condition that needs help?

If you have one of the minor discomforts such as heartburn or constipation, and you're concerned enough about it to be uncomfortable, or if it's upsetting your normal daily activities, then go see your doctor and lay it all out for him. Remember, you're going to tell him exactly what you feel, how it affects you, where it hurts, and if you're under any stress.

If you have I.B.S. and want a second opinion when your first doctor gives you a polite run-a-round, by all means get another doctor's evaluation. The key to taking some action against I.B.S. is when any of the noted conditions cause you problems and upset your normal daily routine. Then be sure to go see your doctor to rule out any of the more serious diseases of the gastrointestinal tract, and see if the physician has any :olid suggestions to fight your condition.

Now, you have a good overview of the general I.B.S. situation and how it can affect you and how to know if you have it. Let's move on to the individual conditions that are called I.B.S. and look at each of them in more detail.

4
GAS, BLOATING & FLATULENCE

STOMACH GAS IS ONE of the minor afflictions that everyone suffers from at one time or another. It's uncomfortable, nagging and a nuisance. When it becomes more than that, and when it happens once a day or every time after you eat, it's more than a nuisance, it's a medical problem that you should take care of.

Gas is one of the conditions that plague I.B.S. patients. What most people think of as gas on their stomach is simply ambient air that they have swallowed while eating, drinking, and sometimes during running or hard physical exercise. A lot of people eat quickly, gulp their food, and in the process intake large quantities of air.

Your stomach can't digest air. It floats around usually searching for the highest area to collect in. If you're standing up, that means the air goes to the top of your stomach near the valve that opens into the esophagus.

Stomach gas has been scientifically evaluated and found to be mainly nitrogen and oxygen with a little bit of carbon dioxide. That's the same description of our atmosphere.

Which led those researchers to figure out that the gas in your stomach is little more than ambient air around your dinner table, and it's now in your belly because you put it there.

The obvious answer to problems of stomach gas is not to gulp down all that air in the first place. Which means to eat slowly, chew your food well, don't gulp, try pointedly not to take in a big mouthful of air as you swallow your food.

You can get air into your stomach other ways: by drinking carbonated beverages and beer, by eating meringues, souffles, whipped cream and all kinds of light and fluffy foods. These make up a minor amount of the total of your air intake.

THE OLD BELCH

Yes, everyone belches now and then. Many people learn to conceal the fact behind a hand or by turning, or by exercising some kind of stomach control that lets the belch out in a more controlled and quieter fashion.

In some countries, a good loud belch after a meal is the best compliment to the cook that you can give.

Some people think that they belch a lot more than most folks and they have some sort of dangerous stomach malady that is relieved and made to feel much better with a raucous belch now and then.

Take it from us, there is no "cause" of belching linked with any stomach ailments or disease. Belching is almost

100% the product of that air you have swallowed while eating, drinking or playing.

How to relieve your belching? Easy. Stop swallowing that air when you eat. Take a moment and study yourself as you eat your next meal. Are you rushing a bit so you can plunge into a conversation gap? Do you try to mix your food with air before you swallow it? Do you slurp and suck liquids through a straw and along with the liquid get a lot of bubbles of air?

The hardest job some gastroenterologists have is to convince their "gas pains" patient that he is his own worst perpetrator of the cause of his burping. As a test, try to keep your mouth glued shut for the next two hours. Don't eat, don't drink, don't yawn, and above all, don't swallow any air.

If you have a history of burping, you probably won't be able to keep your mouth sealed shut for that long. If you can hold out for the two hours, evaluate the results. Did you burp during that time? Did your burping slow and even stop?

This closed mouth routine can often convince a person with gas pains that he can do something to help himself.

WHAT IF THE GAS WON'T COME UP?

At least belching relieves the gas problem. What happens when the gas doesn't want to cooperate and belch up and out of your gut? That can be a problem. Part of the problem is the gas isn't in your stomach anymore.

Doctors call this situation bloating. Much to the surprise of researchers half a century ago, they found out that a person with bloating had about the same amount of gas in his belly as the person who had no bloating and complained of no pains.

Even knowing this, doctors find that people really do have a problem with bloating. One theory is that some patients have hypersensitive bowels. They tend to overreact to the normal amount of gas in the intestines.

We've moved out of the stomach now and into the small intestine. Here the walls of the intestines are supposed to gently push everything downstream. When they encounter this gas, for some reason and in some people, the intestine seems to rebel. It goes into spasms and instead of pushing the fluids downstream, it shoves them upstream back toward the stomach.

Soon the two flows collide and we have a real stoppage, if even for only a few minutes. This is what causes the bowel to swell and that makes the pain. Those who have sensitive small intestines like this usually are also hypersensitive to pain, reacting much stronger than a normal person would in the same situation.

Many patients say they feel more pain after a normal sized or a large meal. One logical answer here would be to eat several smaller meals a day, say six, instead of three larger ones. This makes many patients feel better, but it plays hob with their normal daily activities. Usually there is no special food that the person is sensitive to, it's just food in general.

The addition of fiber here is of no help to bloating. The contents of the small intestine are in liquid form, so the high fiber doesn't aid. It will help when it gets to the large intestine.

Activity after meals, and before the bloating starts, is a help to some patients. The bowel is a muscle, and all muscles react well to exercise. Resting after eating as an aid to digestion is one of those old wive's tales with little value.

Wish you could belch to relieve the pressure? You probably can't. The gas is beyond the stomach and outside of the normal belching area.

DRUG HELP?

Yes, there are some. Anti-gas medications won't help because the problem is beyond the stomach area and we're dealing with muscles. Some drugs can help some people, but with others it's a trial and error situation.

One help is the anticholinergic group of drugs. They work to suppress the cholinergic nerves that drive your muscles and help your organs to perform. By taking one of these drugs, it very well may suppress the action of those rebelling muscles in your intestine, but it also can do the same kind of suppression to other areas of your body.

For example, such anticholinergic drugs could dry out your mouth, your vision might blur, it might become extremely difficult to urinate and your brain could start to shut down and you'd be so sleepy you might not be able to stay awake. These side effects stop many bloating victims from using these types of drugs. Other people use them in small doses and put up with the side effects. For some people, they simply don't help much.

Some gastroenterologists use the drug metoclopramide which increases the bowel action and may work toward smoothing out the muscle spasms that cause the trouble.

Gaining more acceptance as a medication for bloating is the use of a mild antidepressant drug such as ten milligrams of Doxepin. This dosage is so low it couldn't have any effect at all on a truly depressed person. However the slight effect on the sufferer of bloating is often enough to help relieve some of the condition and the pain.

Many doctors now use mild antidepressants to relieve conditions that involve muscle spasms such as low back pain, tension headaches, and whiplash.

So, what to do about bloating? Work closely with your doctor to find out what's causing the spasms, and try to find some medication or exercise that might help relieve it.

FLATULENCE

Passing air, breaking wind, farting, all mean about the same thing, that embarrassing need to equalize the pressure inside and outside of your bowels. Everyone does it. Flatulence is a normal human bodily activity that spares no one. Most people learn how to control it, to do it in the bathroom or hold it until they are alone. Others can't do this.

What's normal? Most individuals generate from three-quarters of a pint to two quarts of gas each day. Many individuals pass air from ten to twelve times a day. Some as much as twenty times. Those who are strict vegetarians pass air many more times than that due to their diet.

This gas is not from that swallowed air we talked about before. Little of that air gets into the lower bowel. The gas there is generated by bacteria that live and work in your lower intestine. Almost all microorganisms produce gas as they do their work.

The food we eat has something to do with how much gas our gut produces. High on the list of the worst gas producers are foods that contain carbohydrates. Your healthy, hard working small intestine breaks down only a small fraction of carbos. Most are passed along to the large intestine where the bacteria there take care of the rest of the digestion. The more they work, the more gas they produce, the more you pass air.

The worst foods for producing gas are beans, peas and peanuts, bran, oats, white wheat flour and milk and other products made with or from milk. Those carbos are simply the hardest to digest, and produce the most flatulence.

MILK CAN HURT YOU

Milk can be a villain? You bet. Man is the only animal where the adult drinks milk. Mother's milk is for babies. Cow's milk is for calves. By the time a human child reaches the age of twelve or thirteen, his body's ability to digest milk starts to be weaned out of his system.

This is called lactase deficiency and many adults have it, and some children. Lactase is a digestive enzyme secreted in the small intestine. It's main job is to digest lactose, the sugar in milk.

When a person becomes an adult, the pattern is set. Some 20 percent of Caucasians from Northern Europe and England can't digest milk. All other ethnic groups have a 75 percent lactase deficiency by the time they are adults.

Chances are that milk could be causing your problems.

If so, when you drink milk the lactose goes right through your stomach and small intestine untouched and hits your colon. The bacteria there have a party multiplying and fermenting the lactose. This will quickly produce lots of gas, which can lead to cramps and often a spate of diarrhea.

You have three choices if milk causes you digestive problems. You can simply eliminate all milk and other dairy products from your diet. With milk used in so many cooked dishes and pastries, this is all but impossible.

You can try to get your calcium through the use of yogurt and cheese. These have already been fermented and you may be able to eat these without any trouble.

If you must cut out all milk products, take a calcium supplement. Calcium carbonate is best, about one gram a day.

FOODS AND FLATULENCE

Yes, some foods really give your flatulence a field day.

Here are a few of those said by experts to cause the most gas in the lower intestine and the most flatulence:

☐ Dried apricots, bananas, beans, bran, Brussels sprouts, carrots, all dried fruit, milk and dairy products, oat bran, onions, peas, raisins and wheat germ.

Foods with the least flatulence consequences:

☐ Eggs, soft drinks, water, red meat, fish, gelatin desserts, chicken and turkey.

ANY DRUGS THAT WORK?

Sorry, not even our big pharmaceutical companies can come up with a drug that will eliminate flatulence. About the closest thing to that is the lowly charcoal pill.

This is a product that's been in drug and health food stores for years and it works. This is activated charcoal, which means it's been heated and then steamed so it has a rough surface. This product grabs almost anything it comes in contact with. It soaks up a lot of the gas in the gut and carries it right out when it's discharged. It works. If you have a serious flatulence problem, try the activated charcoal for a week and see if it makes any difference.

One caution. If you're on medication don't use the charcoal while the drug is in your system. The charcoal will soak up the drug as well and you won't get the benefit from it you need.

The good side: Activated charcoal is over the counter with no prescription needed. Long term use will cause you no problems, it has no side effects and it's impossible to overdose on it.

Flatulence? You can control it to some extent with charcoal tablets and your choices of food. You'll never eliminate it. The best thing is to do all you can to prevent it, then learn how to camouflage what's left and get on with your life.

5
HEARTBURN & YOUR ESOPHAGUS

NOBODY IS GOING TO TELL YOU that heartburn is all in your mind. Almost every living human has experienced it now and again. Estimates put the total number of people in the U.S. who suffer heartburn at least once a month at over forty million. So, you are not alone, and a lot of folks are working on the problem.

Heartburn is most often described as a burning sensation in the middle of the chest. It comes after eating. Other people say it also can be a burning in the abdomen, pressure in their chest and acid from the stomach backing up into their throat.

A WORD OF CAUTION

Since heartburn causes a burning and pain in the chest, it is easy to confuse it with angina or an actual heart attack. Before medical people understood heart attacks, the pain in the chest and subsequent deaths of many people, was called acute indigestion.

President Warren Harding died on August 2, 1923, two years into his first term in office of...."acute indigestion."

Since indigestion or heartburn is so similar in feeling to a real heart attack or angina, it is always highly important to rule out the chance of a heart attack.

Don't simply assume that you are having heartburn. There are a few ways to make sure it's heartburn. Even doctors have trouble sometimes telling the difference so you will, too. If you or a friend has a bad case of heartburn, remember these points:

- ☐ Heart attack pain is severe. If your chest pain is troublesome, hurts a little, but doesn't make you screech in pain or yell at your spouse, it's probably heartburn. Men sometimes say it isn't a severe pain, more of an intense pressure or squeezing feeling. Again, if it is severe it could be a heart attack.

- ☐ Heartburn will go away in five to ten minutes. A heart attack pain lasts and lasts. That's the big difference.

- ☐ The pain could be angina which is a heart condition that causes pain in the chest and means you could have a heart attack down the road. This isn't a 911 emergency, but you should talk to your doctor about it the first time it happens.

Not trying to scare you, but be sure you know the difference between the feeling of heartburn and the long lasting and severe pain of a heart attack.

If you show any of the other symptoms of a heart attack, give your doctor a call at once.

ON WITH HEARTBURN

Heartburn happens when your lower esophageal sphincter, let's call it LES, slips open and those powerful stomach acids leak upward into your esophagus. That strong acid irritates your esophagus, and it hurts like crazy.

Why are some people troubled by heartburn and others who eat the same foods pain free? Some types of individuals are more prone to heartburn than others. Anything that creates pressure on the stomach can do the trick. The pressure can force those gastric juices and acid past a weak LES into your esophagus and you have heartburn.

What causes pressure on the stomach? Pregnancy is one of the big ones, but it usually takes nine months to relieve this pressure. Tight fitting clothes with cinched up belts can cause that pressure and heartburn. Even straining to burp or to have a bowel movement, or even on some exercise machine or climbing a mountain, could cause pressure on your stomach and result in heartburn. Another cause of that pressure can be too much weight.

Night time heartburn can occur when you eat a lot before going to bed and then lie down. Your flat position allows more of your stomach contents to flow toward your LES and put pressure on it and if it's weak, the back flow can take place. Even bending over and squatting after a meal can help to give you heartburn.

WHAT TO DO

Your gastroenterologist will call your heartburn acid reflux. Reflux simply means to "flow back." We often divide heartburn into three do-it-yourself treatment parts.

PART 1

What we try to do here is to help you keep the contents of your stomach in your stomach. That way you have no heartburn. To do that:

Try to eat slower. Listen to TV as you eat, talk about a favorite topic, simply slow down the rate at which you eat. This will help in several ways.

After you eat keep your body upright so you don't give that food slurry a chance to move up to your weak LES valve and have the chance to reflux. Try to keep upright for 3 hours after you eat. This means no two o'clock afternoon nap after your lunch. It also means you shouldn't eat anything substantial for three hours before you go to bed. Forget that late night snack.

The third way to help, especially if you have night heartburn, is to put 6" blocks under the legs at the head of your bed. This will elevate the upward angle of your whole body and force any stomach acid to flow uphill even to get in contact with your LES valve.

PART 2

Determine what foods loosen that LES valve. This varies from person to person, but there are a few foods that some people try to avoid to help their LES valve. These include fruit juices, spices and onions.

The major culprits most people should avoid are alcohol, coffee, fats, peppermint and spearmint candies and chocolate. Yes, we know, we've just described some of the major joys of life. Sorry. You might want to test them and see which avoidance will help you.

To do this use the scientific approach. Use the principal of the single differential. That means drop out one food or drink at a time from your diet for a month, and see if it helps your heartburn. If it doesn't move on to another food or drink to test, but start using the first one that didn't matter. Work through your list of foods this way, and find those particular ones you can tolerate and those that you can't.

Smoking, while not a food, will help to loosen your LES valve, too. Use the no smoking month as another test to see if it is a factor. Antihistamines can also help weaken that LES valve, but when you need the antihistamine medication, you'll probably use it to get rid of a more pressing problem.

PART 3

Keep your stomach as acid free as possible, and strengthen that LES valve.

Strengthening can be a problem. Foods high in protein will do it, if you can get them without a high fat content.

The next move to make is what you've probably been doing all along, to neutralize that stomach acid as much as possible. Do this by taking any of the over the counter antacids. Two tablespoons is a good dosage, even though the label may suggest less. Take it one and three hours after a meal and again just before you go to bed.

Try all of these helps on a continual basis, be consistent. The idea is to stop your heartburn for at least six weeks to give your esophagus a chance to heal. Then if a little acid leaks upward from time to time, it won't hurt your esophagus as much and you won't be bothered with excessive heartburn.

SOMETHING STUCK IN YOUR THROAT?

Now and again a person tries to swallow something and it doesn't work quite right and he or she thinks that there is something stuck in the throat. By "throat" most people really mean the esophagus.

Most of these problems are not problems at all. Sometimes a hard piece of food will scratch the esophagus going down and that can produce the same feeling that there's something stuck down there.

Try a sip of water. If it goes down all right, push the test and try a well chewed bite of food. Chances are what seemed to be stuck in there really isn't stuck at all.

If something actually is stuck in your esophagus and nothing will go down, it's time to get to your doctor quickly. Call and make sure he's at the office, then have someone drive you there without any delay.

BEYOND HEARTBURN

If you have serious heartburn over an extended period of time, the acid reflux from the stomach can adversely affect the lining of the esophagus. What it does is to change. Usually it's made up of squamous cells, but after a continual influx of stomach acid, the cells can change to glandular types. These glandular cells are more like those in the stomach or the intestinal lining.

This problem is called Barrett's esophagus and it's caused by long term acid attacking your esophagus lining. These new cells can make your heartburn much worse. That's because they can secrete acid themselves directly into the esophagus. Before long this can cause your esophagus to develop an ulcer.

Barrett's esophagus also means that the patient is now in an increased danger of developing cancer of the esophagus. If you have Barrett's esophagus you'll have to get regular checkups by your doctor and a gastroenterologist will have to examine you once a year with a long tube down your esophagus that has a lens on it so the doctor can determine if any cancer is present.

The best way to avoid getting Barrett's esophagus is to treat your heartburn and get rid of that stomach acid as fast as you can.

AFTER HOME TREATMENT FOR HEARTBURN

Many doctors instruct their heartburn patients in the three step home treatment program and never see them again. Home treatment will work in most of the cases without a resort to any other type of program.

If the patient comes back and still has the heartburn problem, the next step your doctor probably will take will be with some prescription drugs.

Two of the favorite drugs are Tagamet and Zantac which simply shut off the production of stomach acids. If the acid isn't in the stomach, it can't back up into your esophagus and cause you pain. That's the whole idea with these H-2 blockers, and they are successful in some 95% of the cases.

The main purpose of the acid block is to keep the stomach acids out of the esophagus for long enough to let the tube heal so it won't be so hypersensitive the next time a little stomach acid does work up into it.

IF DRUGS DON'T DO THE TRICK

For those patients who don't respond to the drugs, there is a call on their gastroenterologist who has several more resources and methods to find out why you keep getting heartburn.

One of them is the Berstein test. This requires a tube be put through your nose into your esophagus. He or she will then test your esophagus with salt water or acid to get your reaction.

Another diagnostic tool the doctor can use is the endoscope. This is a soft, flexible tube with fiber-optics and small clever attachments so he can view the inside of your esophagus, take pictures of it, even snip off samples for later research.

If he can't find a good way to make your esophagus well, it may lead to surgery, which we don't want to talk about in this book.

That's it for your heartburn. It can be simply and easily taken care of with some home remedies, or it can lead to serious bouts with more doctors, surgeries and even cancer. Take care of that heartburn, now.

6
NAUSEA & VOMITING

NAUSEA AND VOMITING are two of the most hated words in the whole world. Not because they're bad words, but because of the total and completely terrible feelings that they bring to their victims.

A man said one time, when he was feeling totally nauseous, that he wanted to die rather than live through the terrible upset. A few minutes later he began to vomit and when his stomach was empty but the retching continued, he moaned that he felt so awful he was afraid he wasn't going to die.

This is one of those maladies that we've all had and know about and hope to stay away from. Thousands of people won't step foot on a boat because they're afraid they'll get seasick—even on a calm lake.

Some victims of severe vomiting think that they're going to die. This rarely happens unless the vomiting is a part of something like radiation poisoning.

It takes a lot for the average person to call or go see a doctor when he or she is vomiting. The usual complaint is that the person can keep nothing down. The advice here is simply don't eat or drink anything until you feel better.

Your body is telling you something. You don't know what it is, and the doctor probably won't know what it is. You've picked up a small bug somewhere, some ugly virus, that doesn't like your last meal.

Remember that even though you feel terrible during and after vomiting, you're in no danger. The average adult can vomit for a day without any serious complications.

Whatever you do, don't try to eat or drink anything. This applies to motion sickness pills such as Dramamine and Marazine. These pills can help prevent you from getting seasick or motion sickness, but once you start to throw up, the pill can't do you much good.

So, the best thing to do for a vomiting stomach is to let it run its course without trying to put any medicine or magic fluids into it. Just be miserable but don't eat or drink anything. Yes, rinse out your mouth after vomiting and retching. This will help get rid of the acid and bile taste. A few chunks of ice to suck on won't hurt a thing, since there's less water in that ice than you'll be swallowing from your own saliva.

Some health experts say that a person should call a doctor after vomiting or retching six times. Why six? Who knows. By that time everything that was in your stomach is now in your sink or toilet bowl and down the drain. If you want a handy number, six works as well as any.

The message here should be clear. For vomiting: don't

take any medicine, don't eat or drink anything, don't do anything that will continue the upset of your stomach.

After six or seven hours of vomiting you'll probably taper off and not have any more retching. At least we hope so. For your first adventure with food after vomiting, give your roiling beast of a stomach a gentle dose of sugar in the form of a soft drink. Be sure to use the real sugar type, not diet. Best to open the drink (7-Up is the preferred drink for bad stomachs on fishing boats) and let it come to room temperature and de-fizz itself for a half hour or so. You don't want the carbonation, you want the sugar.

A cola or any other soft drink is easy to digest, and that's what you want to get your old gut back on the road to becoming normal. Water isn't as good simply because it doesn't have to be digested. It's absorbed quickly and gives your digestive juices nothing to do to start your stomach on the road back to normal.

WAIT IT OUT

Nearly half of all vomiting problems last for less than six hours and ninety percent of them will be history after twelve hours.

So, you've finished with the upchucking and feel that you'll starve if you don't eat something. Wrong. Any normal adult can go one or even two days without a stick of food and suffer no more than a few hunger pangs. What that means is don't force yourself to eat to "keep up your strength" if you're still feeling a little queasy and would rather not face mashed potatoes with drippings gravy, greasy French fries and a big bowl of chili.

AGAIN, WAIT IT OUT

Most of the time your flu bug or bad dinner or un-named virus that caused your vomiting will run its course and in a few hours you'll feel much better. Often nausea makes you feel terrible, but after one or two vomiting sessions you'll feel much better. Strange, right, but true.

If you continue to vomit and retch ten or twelve times, you should get on the phone to your doctor. Tell him or her what the problem is and hope for a quick return call.

If you have a steady abdominal pain when you vomit, be sure to call your doctor at once. This could be something more serious such as an ulcer, gallstones or a kidney stone. These pains are severe and you'll want to run, not walk to your nearest medical specialist. There could even be some appendicitis involved here if the pain is that low. While vomiting isn't a typical symptom of a bad appendix, it could be. Don't take any chances and contact your doctor.

NAUSEA AND THE QUEASIES

Sometimes you can get nausea and never vomit. This is a tough one because you soon wish you could vomit so you would feel better.

There are a lot of different causes for this type of nausea. It might be a slight viral infection not strong enough to induce vomiting. It could be an emotional shock, a surprise, a tragedy, some visual problem, motion sickness from a car or boat, hormone changes and even pregnancy. One Broadway actor of a fine reputation worried so much about his night performance that he threw up twenty minutes to curtain time every night.

You've heard about pregnant women who eat crackers to fight morning sickness. Works. Dry toast will do the same thing. Both of these make your stomach produce its acid and enzymes to start digesting the dry things it discovers inside itself. This is a first step to feeling better.

It also encourages your stomach to work, and move the food along to the small intestine. Here that dose of sugar will help. It can be in a soft drink, or a few spoonfuls of honey or molasses can also do the job.

For most of us, an upset stomach is something to live through. Vomiting is a part of life and it takes something rather serious before we call our doctor. Best idea is to do nothing for your vomiting and nausea, and most of the time they will simply fade away and you can get back into action. You'll "feel it in your gut" when you need to call your doctor.

7
EMPTY STOMACH PAINS

HOW CAN YOUR STOMACH HURT when nothing's in it? Answer, easy. The reason is that there is always something in your stomach. It might not be food or drink, but the lining, the muscles, the nerve endings, the enzymes and the acids are always there.

Should you worry about stomach pains? Everyone has some minor clitches and clatches in the belly now and again. Most of them are minor and temporary and you forget about them. Don't dash off to see your doctor at every little cramp or pain. For the more severe, longer lasting pains, keep on using your common sense, ask yourself some questions and see if there is an easy answer you can come up with.

If a stomach pain persists and there are other symptoms as well that trouble you, by all means go see your doctor. Better to be safe than dead.

ACID PAINS

When your stomach hurts when it's empty, it almost always is the result of acid, some drug you've taken or some other irritant. We've talked about the strong acids that the stomach secretes, but we also know that the stomach lining protects the stomach from those same acids.

The acids can cause pain in there if there is some problem or disease in the stomach. So remember that stomach pain can be a symptom of something much more serious.

DRUG PAINS?

Yes, a whole group of drugs can cause pains to your empty stomach. Probably the one that does the most damage even today is the common aspirin. When an aspirin goes into an empty stomach, it literally burns a hole in the outer lining. That can cause you pain. This hole is not deep and it will heal within a few days, but it does some damage. This takes place even for those people who are not sensitive to aspirin.

If you need to take aspirin, the safest way is to mash it up in a spoon with another spoon until it's a fine powder. Then either dissolve the powder in water and take it with a glass of water, or take the powder dry and then drink a glass of water. Result: no hole in your stomach lining.

Why take aspirin at all when there are other pain relievers advertised heavily that don't irritate your stomach? The answer is that aspirin still does more. Aspirin relieves your pain and it also inhibits prostaglandins, which researchers feel are partly responsible for the pain of arthritis, bursitis, muscle injuries and menstrual cramps. So aspirin still has its place.

You can also take acetaminophen, that is trademarked as Tylenol and Datril. To knock out pain of fever and minor pains, aspirin is still just as good as Tylenol despite what the TV ads say.

What pain relievers do is dull your brain to the pain, making you feel better. The pain is still there, you just don't feel it.

Other drugs for pain include the ibuprofens such as Advil and Nuprin. Ibuprofen is a good pain reliever and less irritating to the stomach than aspirin. Prescription pain relievers will also affect the stomach. These include Naprosyn, Indocin and Anaprox.

Some antibiotics can cause you stomach pain as well. If this happens, talk to your doctor and see if you can get another antibiotic that will be easier on your stomach.

What else can give you stomach pains? Lots of things including iron pills, potassium supplements, even alcohol, caffeine and nicotine.

If your stomach comes up painful, the first thing to think about is if you have taken any pain pills or other drugs or medications that may be doing the dirty work.

WHAT ABOUT AN ULCER?

The worst villain in the empty stomach pain department is the problem of an ulcer. One of the symptoms of an ulcer is if you have pain on an empty stomach or more than two hours after eating. Your doctor will want to know about this one. Rule out medications first, then think ulcer.

Most doctors find that only about one quarter of those patients with typical ulcer symptoms turn out to have the problem.

So, can you do some self evaluating on your own stomach pain? Glad you asked. If you have empty stomach pain, ask yourself these questions:

1. Does eating something or taking an antacid help relieve the pain?

   Usually antacids and food will relieve stomach pain caused by acid. If one or both of these relieve your stomach pain, there's a chance you do have an ulcer. The trouble is, both antacids and food also can eliminate pain from other stomach ills such as gastritis and non-ulcer dyspepsia. This isn't enough evidence to say you have an ulcer.

2. Are there some foods that make your empty stomach pain worse?

   Some say that fruit juices and spices make the pain worse. Then eliminate such foods from your diet and some of the pain will vanish. However, many people are intolerant to many foods, so this doesn't help figure out if you have an ulcer.

3. Do you have any other symptoms?

   Non-ulcer dyspepsia can lead to belching, nausea, bloating, heartburn, a feeling of fullness and vomiting. So this could be your problem. However these symptoms also occur sometimes with ulcers, so again it isn't a reliable judge about an ulcer you might have.

4. Does aspirin make your stomach hurt?

   If so, it's an indicator you may have an ulcer. Over two thirds of ulcer victims have a sensitivity to aspirin.

5. Do you have stomach pain at night?

   Your stomach secretes most of its acid about 2 AM. If you get empty stomach pain then, it could be an indicator of an ulcer. Again it's a weak clue because almost all stomach diseases and many stomach upsets produce night time stomach pain.

WHAT NEXT?

If you think you have an ulcer, see your doctor and lay out the answers to the above five questions. Actually it doesn't matter a great deal what your problem is: an ulcer, gastritis or non-ulcer dyspepsia. The treatment for all three is exactly the same.

HOME TREATMENT

In this case you can start the same treatment the doctor would tell you to do.

1. If you're smoking, stop cold turkey. Eliminate all stomach irritants such as caffeine and aspirin. This includes coffee and cola drinks.

2. Use antacids, two teaspoons full one hour after eating, again three hours after eating and at bedtime.

3. Maintain this treatment for seven days. You should be better after a week and pain free in a month. If after seven days your symptoms are the same, see your doctor.

8
FULL STOMACH PAINS

Lᴇᴛ's sᴀʏ ɪᴛ's ʏᴏᴜʀ ʙɪʀᴛʜᴅᴀʏ. For dinner you're having all three of your favorite entrees, plus six side dishes, a glass of wine, delicious hot soft bread sticks, gobs of homemade strawberry jam, and then three kinds of dessert to choose from or you can have them all. Not bad, right?

Not until you roll away from the table, your hands covering your stomach as you waddle across the room to the sofa and flake out full length on your back.

"Got a bellyache," you tell your spouse.

True. The major cause of pain in the stomach when you're eating or finished, and up to an hour and a half or so afterwards, is simply gluttony. You ate too much. Your stomach is fully extended, you sucked in two pints of air with your food and that takes up more stomach space.

Then you were so excited and pleased with the birthday dinner and the glorious presents that you didn't bother to chew your food well enough. That means your stomach now must secrete more enzymes and acids to break down those larger food chunks which puts more pressure in the already filled sack.

Miserable.

Over-stuffing your stomach is the number one reason for a painful stomach when it has food in it. Figures. Over-stuffing usually takes place during a long meal, such as at a holiday. The stomach needs twenty minutes before it can signal the brain that it's full and then your brain lets you know quickly.

How not to get that over-stuffed feeling? The most obvious is simply eat less. Another better help is to eat slower. You tend to eat less and to gulp down less air when you eat slower and chew your food better. This will also reduce the amount of stomach fluids needed and further keep from "filling you up."

Sorry there aren't any medicines, pills or potions to help you get over an over stuffed stomach. The only thing that will do it is time. In two hours, you'll be feeling great again.

SMALL STOMACH, LARGE MEAL

Sometimes a person will simply have a small stomach. This could come about when a person is dieting. After a week or two of eating two small meals a day the stomach will simply shrink in size. Then if you go off your diet and try for a pound and a half T-Bone steak with all the side dishes and two desserts, you won't be able to get half way through before you feel "full."

This doesn't happen often, but it can be a problem for dieters who go overboard by not eating, then surge back.

Then there is the person with a "nervous stomach." Here the muscles in the stomach contract and jump around for no specific reason. When this happens, the stomach tends to shrink and won't accept as much food.

This nervous stomach is probably tied to some kind of reaction to stress. It's psychosomatic, but terribly real just the same. Different people react in different ways to stress. You should know what your physical reactions are when you get stressed out.

Some people vomit. Others get angry and scream and yell. Some simply curl up within themselves and vanish from the problem area or the problem family members. Know what your psychosomatic reaction is to high stress. That way you can handle it better, even plan ahead for it.

If your reaction is a nervous stomach, there probably won't be much you can do about it. Try to control the cause of the stress. Trying to eat several smaller meals a day could help.

To get rid of the root problem, the stress, you'll have to make some drastic changes in your life style. Few people want to, or are able to, do this. They would rather have a slightly stressed out stomach than quit their job, move to Tahiti, and take a second spouse twenty years younger than themselves.

One way to help relieve a stressed stomach problem is to try to relax before a meal. Some people find a beer and good conversation with friends helps. Others will go on a casual walk in the woods or along a stream. Some exercise until they sweat, or read two chapters in a good book they're working on. Whatever you can do to get relaxed and in a pleasant state, will help to relax your stressed stomach as well, and you'll have more chances of eating a regular meal.

If nothing works, it's back to the five or six meals a day, or at least two large snacks between your usual three a day where you're eating less than you should.

For an overloaded stomach, you probably won't need to go see your doctor unless it becomes a serious problem and you begin to lose weight. If all else fails, make an appointment and try for an unbiased opinion about your gastric problems.

UNRELATED, BUT CAUSALLY LINKED

When your stomach is full, it signals your gallbladder to produce more bile that you need for digestion. The tie in with a full stomach is tenuous, but it fits neatly enough for this purpose.

You could get another abdominal pain about this time that is unrelated to the amount of food you've eaten. There could be pain from gallstones.

Large gallstones don't bother you, they simply sit and

grow slightly larger in the midst of your bile. The tiny stones are washed right down through the bile ducts and you or your stomach never know it.

The problems come when a stone just a little too large to pass all the way through the bile duct gets flooded downstream and stuck part way through.

Talk about pain. You'll know it. A stone stuck in the bile duct will give you screaming pain or perhaps just a whimper depending on the size and exactly where it is. Often after less than an hour or up to four hours, the stone works its way through the bile duct and the pain goes away. The stone might go out the far end of the duct or be jolted back into the gallbladder. With the intense pain, some patients have a bout with nausea and vomiting.

Most of the gallstones that start through the bile ducts make it. It's an exception when a gallstone becomes so lodged in the bile duct that it takes surgery to remove it.

To help prevent gallstones, keep a slim profile. Fat people have more trouble this way than those slender ones in good physical condition.

If you get one of the whammer painful gallstone attacks and go see a doctor, you'll get pain medication first. If the medication is good for four hours, usually the attack by the gallstone is over by the time the pain medicine fades out.

9
DIARRHEA

DIARRHEA IS A MALADY that everyone knows about. It can strike with amazing speed after a bit of tainted food is eaten, it can last for days or it can be over and done with in a half hour. Diarrhea is usually described as an extreme loose and watery stool or when a person's bowel movements become too frequent.

Most bouts with diarrhea require no medical attention. They are sometimes the body getting rid of a problem, such as a light case of food poisoning, that clears up by itself in a few hours. There are several other reasons why people get diarrhea, including nervous tension and it can be a symptom of some far more serious and even life threatening diseases.

If your situation continues for a matter of hours or even days, it could be something that's more complicated.

If your diarrhea is chronic and lasts for weeks, it could be a sign of a serious illness such as colitis or some form of intestinal cancer. It might mean that a parasite has taken up permanent residency in your bowels. For either of these problems, you need prompt medical attention.

What is called acute diarrhea is less severe and could last a half hour or two or three days. It is almost always caused by your small intestine not absorbing the nutrients or the water in it and may be secreting more than it's absorbing. This is why you'll have heavy, watery stools that shoot right through you like a Fourth of July rocket.

Diarrhea can also be an indictor of a food intolerance or an allergy.

For most of us, an attack of diarrhea means we have had a touch of food poisoning or an infection from a vicious virus or bacteria. For adults this is a discomforting inconvenience, but for a baby or infant, diarrhea can be fatal. Infants are more susceptible to the problems that diarrhea can cause. Over any extended length of time, it prevents food from being utilized by the body, can cause dehydration no matter how much liquid is given, and can mean a quick weight loss, malnutrition and possible starvation.

These problems with children are especially severe among the U.S. poor and those in the South. In the Third World nations, almost five million infants and children die of diarrhea every year.

WHAT DO THOSE BUGS DO DOWN THERE?

When you get a touch of food poisoning, for example, the bad bacteria, like Salmonella, give off toxins that stick to the lining of the small intestine. The cells in the lining don't like this and start trying to neutralize them with secretions. The cells gush out much more fluid than they normally absorb and the net result is more outflow than absorption.

This mixture is then quickly passed down the small intestine into the colon where it is ushered right on through and you have diarrhea.

A SELF-CHECK FOR YOUR DIARRHEA

First, understand that diarrhea is not a disease, it's a condition and a common symptom of many different problems and diseases. Some are extremely serious, so you should know what kind of diarrhea you have so you can get medical help if you need it. No, it's not all that hard, and any adult with average intelligence (reported to be at about the 7th grade level) can do the task quite well. Answer these questions:

1. How long have you had diarrhea?

   It's probably acute diarrhea if you've had it less than a week. It should be finished soon, and could be already gone. A mild touch of food poisoning could be over within an hour after you eat. Then you'll feel much better.

   If your problem recurs and is sporadic, it could be irritable bowel syndrome. This is true if the diarrhea is a result of stress and is interspersed with bouts of constipation. A good guideline is that if your diarrhea lasts for ten days or more, make an appointment to see your doctor.

2. What do your stools look like?

    Are you sure it's diarrhea? Occasional frequent movements, three or four a day, might not be diarrhea. To be diarrhea your stool must be watery, almost liquid, sometimes explosive exiting, and much more voluminous than usual.

3. Is there any blood on or in your stool?

    Blood on the outside of the more solid parts of your stool probably only means that you have some bleeding from hemorrhoids near your anus. This is not diarrhea. If you have chronic diarrhea that's bloody with the blood mixed into much of the stool, it's more serious. It could be a parasite infection or even a cancer somewhere in your digestive tract. See your doctor at once.

4. Do you have a fever?

    Usually there's not much of a rise of temperature with most types of diarrhea. If you have a rise in your temperature, even if slight and it persists, you could have the flu or it could be an early sign of appendicitis.

Check it out with your doctor to be sure.

5. Been hiking, camping or traveled abroad recently?

    If so, you could have picked up an infection or parasite from the local water or by drinking untreated water from a stream. Parasites that people in other countries get used to and rebuff, can cause a lot of trouble for travelers. If your "foreign" diarrhea lasts for several days, you should see your doctor for some tests.

6. Is it your menstrual time?

    If you have endometriosis or irritable bowel syndrome or both, you also may have diarrhea. Not a lot to do about it but it usually ends when your period ends.

7. Do others around you have diarrhea?

    If people you live with or work with have diarrhea, you may all have developed it from eating the same contaminated food. Has there been a hot-day picnic lately that you attended? Picnics are a classic way to get sick from tainted food.

8. Does your baby or child have diarrhea?

    Breast fed babies have far less diarrhea than those on formula. However if the baby is allergic to cow's milk and the mother drinks milk, the breast milk will also carry the allergic reaction for the baby. Juices such as apple and pear are hard for babies to absorb and may result in diarrhea. If the child's diarrhea is due to a parasite, it may have been contracted in a day school.

9. What drugs are you using?

   Some prescription drugs, some antibiotics, antacids and some laxatives can give you diarrhea. Some drugs for thyroid are culprits too, as well as many of the drugs used for chemotherapy in fighting cancer.

10. Too much alcohol?

    If you drink too much wine, beer or hard liquor you can have diarrhea with no other cause. Since the diarrhea prevents their small intestine from getting any nourishment from their food, many alcoholics can easily become victims of malnutrition.

HOME TREATMENT FOR DIARRHEA

Let's say you have an upset stomach a half hour after eating at a fancy restaurant. Your stomach growls, you have some cramps then you dash for the bathroom and explode all over the bowl. You've had some type of minor tainted food problem. The trouble should pass soon and you'll feel better and have no recurrence. No treatment needed.

Another time you have diarrhea a few hours after eating, but you skip a meal and have no more trouble. This probably means that your bowel is not absorbing the fluids.

Try the six hour system. Six hours after your last movement, try sipping some soft drink with real sugar, not a diet drink. This will give your digestive system some easy to process sugar and see how it does.

If that doesn't cause you any more upset, move on to a banana, some white rice, applesauce and some chamomile herbal tea. Not all at once, of course, but use them as you come back from the brink of any more eruptions.

One small operational hint. If you're having liquid stools, try lying down for a while. Just as gas rises as high as it can, so does liquid move downward as far as possible. If that watery stool gets into your rectum area, you'll need to go again. Lying down will make the liquid stay in your colon longer and give it more chance to absorb some of it, and help reduce your diarrhea.

The World Health Organization has an aid for people in poor nations where diarrhea is epidemic. They use as a first drinking liquid a mixture of a liter of water, which is one quart and one fourth-cup for us, one half teaspoon of salt, one fourth teaspoon of potassium chloride, one half teaspoon of baking soda and four tablespoons of sugar. The sugar is to give the bowel something easy and quick to digest.

This is just as good as a soft drink and a lot less expensive where that's a factor. Check your local laws. Most states restrict the sale of potassium chloride as a prescription item.

Opium is the all time, ages old best drug to treat diarrhea. A tincture of opium would be ideal, but it's so cheap to make that the drug companies don't bother with it.

Your best bet is to look for a paregoric. Two of the brand names are Parapectolin and Parelixir. Some states require a prescription for this product.

Next up is Imodium A-D, now non-prescription and it is an opium derivative. The other old standby is Pepto-Bismol with the liquid working better than the tablets. So you don't get in a panic, remember that Pepto-Bismol will turn your stool black.

Other over the counter products that might work for you are Kaopectate and Donnagel. They have as their job making your watery stool more solid. On some people they work better than on others.

SHOULD YOU GO SEE YOUR DOCTOR?

Most medical people would suggest that you wait at least four days before going to see your doctor. Use the home remedies and if they work you're the winner. This is for an uncomplicated case of diarrhea with no other problems.

If you have a continuing fever or a large volume of stool you might go in earlier. One factor that should make you get a doctor's appointment is if you are losing weight. If you lose five pounds in a few days, and you're not trying to lose weight, make a call and go in. A bloody or blood-blackened stool is another good reason to call for that appointment.

WHAT ABOUT ANTI-DIARRHEA DRUGS?

Yes, there are several on the market and many people rely on them when traveling, especially to Mexico and the less developed countries around the world where sanitation isn't quite perfected.

Even with the use of these drugs, you should be careful about drinking the local water, and eating fruits and vegetables that can't be peeled. This is again in the Third World countries. But even in the western nations you'll find some local bacteria that the residents can tolerate with no trouble, but that will give you a case of the runs in a rush.

Try these drugs when you travel:

☐ Doxycycline is a long acting antibiotic. It will help protect you from bad bugs, but also mean you'll sunburn much easier than normal. No lying on the beach. Sun screen will help you here and with the next drug.

☐ Trimethoprin sulfa. This also is a good antibiotic and you can get a little more sun with this one.

The whole idea of a preventive drug is to take it before you are exposed to the bad bugs and keep taking it during your trip to ward off the little villains. Don't wait until you get diarrhea. It's too late then.

10
CONSTIPATION

MANY DOCTORS DEFINE CONSTIPATION as a person's failure to have a bowl movement for three days or more. That's as good a rule as any, however as we said before, some people need to have two movements a day, and some can go eight or ten days with absolutely no problems whatsoever.

It depends to a large extent on the individual, his or her training, diet and just as important, the amount of exercise that is done.

One and two generations ago doctors spent a lot more time talking with patients about constipation than they do today. We can thank this change on the love affair America has had for the past twenty years with physical fitness, jogging, workout clubs, and the surge in more concern with diet, fats, vegetables and fiber in the diet. Many doctors say they now rarely see any patient under sixty years old who has a complaint about constipation.

WHAT CAUSES CONSTIPATION?

Easy question. Too little fiber in your diet. Too little exercise. There can be some other causes, but these two are the main ones. When put together they almost guarantee bouts of constipation.

Yes, some medications can cause constipation, but when the medication runs its course, the problem is solved. Some people who have excess calcium in their blood and those suffering from low thyroid can also have constipation, but then it becomes an understandable and treatable problem. Pregnant women can also have constipation due to mechanical reasons: just not enough room in there for everyone and everything.

Most constipation comes and goes. It's irritating and bothersome but you soon forget about it and drop back into bad habits again.

HOW TO PREVENT CONSTIPATION

No one knows for sure for everyone, but for most of us the answer is relatively easy: more fiber and more exercise. People confined to bed often have a constipation problem. Exercising is going to mean a slight change in your life style. Some people get up at four in the morning so they can get in their four mile run every day. Others jog after a light lunch, getting in a 40 minute run and a ten minute shower before desk time again.

More people take walks, do treadmills or use exercise machines which have become endemic in our society. Make it a point to get in your exercise daily, or at least three times a week. Knock off a bunch of birds with one stone and do aerobic exercises such as walking, jogging, bicycling, aerobic dancing, anything that keeps you moving constantly for 40 minutes.

Lifting weights is exercise, but not aerobic since you do one rep and rest. Aerobic must be continual to get the work your heart and lungs need.

Fiber is another matter that will take a slight change in your life-style. You like to eat ham and eggs and hash browns for breakfast? Fine, but do it just once a month. In between go for some dry cereal, bran flakes or such, a slice of toast and jam and a couple of dried prunes. Now you're getting some fiber in your diet.

What is fiber? That's the part of fruits, vegetables and grains that your gut can't digest. It's roughage. There is no fiber in meat and dairy products. In fruit juices the fiber has mostly been removed, except some of the new "pulp" orange juice concentrates. So how do you get more fiber in your diet?

The easiest and cheapest way to get more fiber is to simply add unprocessed bran to your foods. It may look a little strange, but it has no taste at all, so that won't stop you. You can sprinkle it on your food or mix it in drinks or even in water. This fiber works by absorbing water in your digestive tract and creates more bulk to push through your innards.

Try a spoonful a day, along with an extra glass of water for that teaspoon of bran. Increase the bran a teaspoon full at a time until you get the regularity you want. Be sure that you drink one glass of water for each extra teaspoon of bran.

Another way is to try to eat more foods with natural fiber in them. Instead of a cheeseburger and fries for lunch, try to go with something with more fiber: a banana, chili with beans, a dinner salad. There's a chapter coming up on diet and a lot of it has to do with more fiber. Take a good long, hard look at that chapter.

Since we're talking about fiber, here are some foods that are high in fiber. We hope that you like some of them and can use them to help control any constipation problem you might have.

Oh, for best colon control you should have from 25 to 30 grams of fiber a day in your diet.

SOURCES OF FIBER

Food	Portion	Grams of Fiber

GRAIN PRODUCTS

Food	Portion	Grams of Fiber
Bagel	1 regular	1.4
Bran from oats	1/3 cup	7.8
Bran flake cereal	2/3 cup	4.6
Bran from corn	1 teaspoon	3.0
Bread, pita whole wheat	1 six inch	2.6
Bread, whole wheat	1 slice	2.2

Brown rice	3/4 cup	2.5
Oatmeal, dry	1/3 cup	2.4
Popcorn, no butter	2 cups	2.6
Rye crackers	2 regular	2.2
Shredded wheat	1 biscuit	3.0
Wheaties (prepared)	1 cup	3.0

VEGETABLES

Broccoli, raw	1/2 cup	1.2
Cabbage, red, raw	1/2 cup	0.7
Carrot, raw	1 medium	2.3
Lettuce, iceberg	1 cup	0.6
Potato with skin	1 medium	3.0
Spinach	1 cup	1.4
Tomato	1/4 medium	0.4

NUTS AND BEANS

Beans, kidney, cooked	1/2 cup	9.0
Beans, pinto, cooked	1/2 cup	9.0
Beans, lima, cooked	1/2 cup	6.6
Beans, 3 bean salad	3/4 cup	8.5
Chick peas, canned	1/2 cup	6.5
Peanut butter, chunky	1 tablespoon	2.6
Peanuts, roasted	1 ounce	1.1

FRUITS

Apple with skin	1 medium	2.8
Banana	1 medium	1.8
Blackberries	1/2 cup	4.5

Cantaloupe	1/4 average	1.3
Dates, dried	5 regular	3.6
Figs, dried	3 regular	9.5
Grapefruit	1/2 regular	0.7
Orange	1 medium	3.1
Orange juice	1 cup	0.5
Pear	1 medium	4.3
Pineapple	1/2 cup	1.0
Raisins	1/4 cup	1.1
Strawberries	1 cup	2.8

TREATING CONSTIPATION

Treating constipation is best done by prevention. Do all you can to get and stay regular through diet. If this doesn't always work there are always the laxatives for temporary relief. If you have constipation for ten days and feel terrible, go to your doctor for some help. You may have more than just constipation.

There are over seven hundred and fifty different cures for constipation on the market. They can be divided into several types. Always use the least caustic and severe type that will do the job for you. They include:

☐ **The bulking type.** These add bulk to your stool to help eject the waste. They include trade names such as Metamucil, Effer-Syllium and Perdiem. These are all made from psyllium seeds and add bulk. Fiber-Con with other ingredients acts the same way.

☐ **Stool softeners.** These are not laxatives as such, but work to keep the stool soft for a better natural passage. An example is Colace.

☐ **Magnesium salts.** This type of laxative increases the fluid in the lower bowel to promote passage. Brand names include Phillips Milk of Magnesia and Haley's M-0.

☐ **Stimulants** increase internal water secretion and contractions to force the stool along. Here we have Ex-Lax and Correctol. Another one, Dulcolax also is a stimulant laxative that works directly on the colon to make it contract.

☐ **Enemas.** More used a generation or two ago, the enema remains as a safe and effective way to treat ordinary constipation. A warm water enema can enlarge the rectum which stimulates the normal action of the colon that starts your defecation.

☐ **Suppositories.** There are several brands on the market. The suppository is one of the best ways to use a laxative. It goes to work at once without having to travel through the whole G.I. tract. It is gentle. It is also a little uncomfortable to use, so it's less likely to become habit forming.

The use of laxatives can become habit forming. The more laxatives are used, the less the body reacts normally to do the same work. The bowels are lazy. If, over time, laxatives do the work for them, they will become sluggish and fail to function even when you do have sufficient bulk in your stool for normal stool passage.

If you need a laxative, use the gentlest of the pack and if you use it more than once, keep a diary of when, so you will realize if you are becoming dependent.

A regular bowel is part of the benefit of regular exercise and a good high fiber diet. Work at both of them. Try to keep your elderly relatives on their feet and active as long as possible. Any kind of exercise, even with a walker or with the aid of an arm holder, is better than sitting in a chair all day or being in bed most of the time.

A final word. Don't skip a meal if you don't have a good reason. Regular eating stimulates the whole G.I. tract and makes everything work better.

11
ANAL ITCHING

ONE OF THE MOST EMBARRASSING **and infuriating** minor maladies of the body is anal itching. Don't shy away, don't be embarrassed, almost everyone has it from time to time, and it can occur for a variety of reasons.

Lack of cleanliness is not a cause of anal itching. In fact this is one area of your body that is best to be let alone. Don't try to over clean it. Warning: never wash your anus with soap. Strange? Not really. The soap can irritate the opening and cause you more pain and problems. Wash lightly without soap and then pat, don't rub, pat dry.

WHY THIS DEVLISH ITCHING?

Anal itching is not one of the complicated irritants of the human body. It's almost always caused by your diet, by stress (yes stress again) or by some minor infection. In this situation, the more you work at cleanliness, the more damage you're going to do in that sensitive area.

What can you do for that wanta-yell-out-loud terrible itching?

First, take a look at your diet. Regular coffee and decaffeinated coffee are the two most common foods that cause anal itching in some individuals. Other drinks that can do it are tea, colas and hot chocolate. These drinks as causes of anal itch are on the rare side, but if you rule out all else, you might consider these drinks as the bad guys.

This one is going to hurt. Dairy products can cause the itching in many people. If that's your problem you'll know it when you cut out all dairy products for two weeks: No milk, cream, cream desserts, ice cream or any of the types of cheeses. This includes main dishes that include cheese such as pizza and all those fine Italian and Mexican foods. If you're going to do the test, do it wholeheartedly. Eat Chinese.

If none of the above have knocked out your anal itching, take a look at your beer and vitamin C intake. So you lay off the beer for two weeks and drop off your vitamin C and see.

MOVING RIGHT ALONG

So your problem wasn't your intake of consumables at all, what does that leave? Maybe a fungus infection. This is one you can treat yourself if that's the problem. Check for itchy pink spots between your legs and around your genitals. If they show up you can be quite sure you have a minor fungus infection.

There are several antifungal creams on the market today: Micatin and another one Lotrimin. Use one of these creams as directed on the package for two weeks. If the itching stops go right on using the cream for two more months to be sure the fungus is eradicated.

If the itching continues after the two weeks, you know you don't have a fungus. Your doctor should take a look at those pink itchy places to be sure they aren't serious.

WHAT DO YOU MEAN IT'S MY #^&($#+&!$) STRESS!

I'm as calm as a pill in a pod, er as cool as a pea in a cucumber. Okay, so I'm a little stressed out.

The big problem is you can't really tell if your anal itching is stress originated until after you check out the other two possibilities. That can take some time.

Stress related problems are not something that you can treat yourself. A good psychologist might be able to help you. One back door, off the floor suggestion might be to try to vent your stress by actually itching somewhere else. Itch your wrist if you're getting edgy at a meeting, or scratch the side of your neck by rubbing it with your fingers. Try rubbing your forehead — someone might believe that you're deep in thought. Sometimes this will substitute for the itching anus. The fine part here is that itching your neck is much more socially acceptable than itching your bottom.

It might be just enough to let you vent your tension and short circuit the anal itching all together.

BUT THE ITCH GOES ON

As you're trying to figure out what is causing this itching, over what might be a two or three month period, you'll want some relief. You can get symptomatic relief with any of the one percent hydrocortisone creams on the market. There are a batch of them including Cortaid, Delacourt and Hytone. Any of these will stop the itching for a time. You may need to use them more than once a day.

Even the hemorrhoid remedies such as Anusol and Preparation H will usually stop the itching. Be careful not to use anything stronger that contains antiseptics or anti-histamines. They can hurt more than the itching does.

CLEANING YOURSELF

After a bowel movement, clean yourself gently with a wet toilet tissue, plain white if possible, or cotton balls. Never clean your anus with soap, and don't use any creams except those we talked about for anti itch. Never, never scrub your anus with one piece of dry toilet paper after another. That can cause you some problems.

Generally when you're trying to clear up an itching situation it's best not to wear panty hose or jockey type shorts. Instead go to the boxer shorts for men and soft, loose cotton panties for women.

If your itch develops into something more serious, such as showing a lump or bleeding or a tear in your skin, that's when you need to see a doctor and let him take over your treatment. He'll know exactly what to do.

12
YOUR DIET & I.B.S.

As MENTIONED BEFORE, Irritable Bowel Syndrome is an umbrella name for several problems that people, mostly under forty years of age and most of those female, have with their gastrointestinal tract.

Specifically these ailments usually include: constipation, diarrhea, stomach pains, heartburn and flatulence. If your I.B.S. involves constipation and flatulence, turn back to those chapters that deal exclusively with those topics and re-read them for an explanation of what's going on and how to deal with it. The same idea holds true for diarrhea, stomach pains and flatulence.

In this chapter we'll go into more detail about how to handle the food and nutritional elements that can have a lot to do with the various I.B.S. conditions.

Our food is the fuel that keeps our body/machine in operation. As with any machine, take away or downgrade the fuel, and you stop or slow down the performance.

In the chapter on how the digestive system works, you saw what a finely tuned manufacturing plant our body is. How it takes almost any food and digests it into chemicals and nutrients that can be absorbed by the small intestine and ushered into the blood where they are utilized.

If you don't give your body the right foods, it's going to malfunction on you somewhere. Your 486, 66 megahertz machine is going to have a lot of glitches in it and simply won't work right or do what you want it to do.

SIX SIMPLE SOLUTIONS

There are six ways that many people can help their G.I. tract to do a better job. All of these are actions that you can take yourself, in fact they are so ingrained that you're the only one who can take care of them. Let's take a look. These six simple solutions to better gastrointestinal health are:

SOLUTION #1: SMOKING—STOP IT

Everyone who smokes must know by this time that it can lead to a number of deadly diseases: lung cancer, pancreatic cancer, emphysema, and a couple of cancers in the G.I. tract. If that kind of argument hasn't pulled your nicotine plug yet, how about this:

- ☐ Smoking makes your chances much higher of developing an ulcer, especially the duodenal ulcer.
- ☐ Smoking aids and abets heartburn. If you get it and you smoke, don't complain about it around us. If your esophageal valve is weak, smoking makes it that much worse.

☐　Smoking can alter your liver's ability to knock out the harmful effects of drugs, alcohol and other toxins.

☐　Smoking lowers your body's ability to absorb nutrients in the food you eat. You're a less efficient eating machine.

How do you stop smoking? Tons of books have been written on the subject and dozens of stop-smoking programs. Pick one and give it a try.

SOLUTION #2: COFFEE—CUT DOWN ON IT

Coffee is the most popular drink in America even though it contains a drug that isn't good for you.

Yes, many of you can't get moving in the morning before you have your first cup of coffee. That's little more than habit, and a habit can be changed. Coffee has not been linked to any deadly disease, yet caffeine is known to be bad for many bodily functions including problems with the male prostate.

When caffeine hits your stomach, it increases the flow of gastric juices. The flavor oils in coffee also stimulate acid secretion in the stomach. You can get an overload of stomach acid in a rush.

Coffee also can mean fewer nutrients are absorbed in the intestine. Coffee drinkers can lose minerals such as magnesium and calcium. It's been proved that coffee also raises your cholesterol level and can make heartburn worse.

Many experts say that two cups of coffee a day won't hurt you, but more than that could have unhealthy effects on you, especially on your GI tract.

SOLUTION #3: ALCOHOL—CUT DOWN

Alcohol is a foreign substance to the body and a poison. Any amount of it does a certain amount of harm. When you drink, alcohol surges through your bloodstream. If your blood-alcohol level is too high, you get arrested for driving while under the influence of a dangerous drug.

Drug? Alcohol is a drug: legal, but still deadly. Drinking to excess is a huge problem in America. Today we have almost nineteen million alcohol abusers. Less than one million of them get any sort of treatment whatsoever.

You swear that you only take a drink now and then and you're not an alcoholic. Fine. Do you drink every day? Can you quit alcohol cold turkey for a month? If your answer was yes to the first question, it probably is no to the second.

Alcohol can damage the intestinal lining which reduces the ability of the small intestine to absorb nutrients. This could lead to ulcers. Alcohol will almost certainly make worse any gastroenterology problems you already have.

SOLUTION #4: SUGAR—CUT DOWN

We all eat too much sugar. On the average every man, woman and kid in the nation eats eighty pounds of sugar a year. That's the average. Many teenagers eat twice their weight in sugar every year.

There are four kinds of sugar, and all turn into the same chemical elements once they get into your digestive tract. The four are sucrose, like table sugar; fructose in fruits, vegetables and corn syrup; glucose or dextrose in honey, other vegetables and corn syrup; and lactose, the sugar in cow's milk.

Unless you live on a farm and grow all of your own food, it's almost impossible to cut much sugar out of your diet. Almost all processed foods contain sugar, even mustard, mayonnaise and salad dressings to say nothing of canned fruits and vegetables.

The purists will wail and moan about sugar, but from a practical level, and unless you want to retreat to that truck gardening farm and raise your own food, there's not much chance to cut out all sugar from your diet.

The best basic approach is to try to limit your optional sugar. We know people who put sugar on sliced tomatoes. You can cut down on sugar in coffee, buy low-calorie, sugar free ice cream, avoid the hyper-sugar breakfast cereals, and take a shot at learning to enjoy foods you don't sugar so much.

The sugar substitutes don't help. Of the four major ones, all have some health problems connected to them that probably are worse than the effects of that much more sugar.

Moderation in sugar is the best way to handle the situation. Cut down on your optional sugar and try to enjoy your food with less sugar out of the bowl on the table. That will help a little.

We all can't be saints.

SOLUTION #5: FAT—CUT DOWN

Most people do better cutting down high fat content foods than they do high sugar content. Mostly this is due to the recent law that required that the contents of food nutrients be printed on every food product packaged and sold. Fats and saturated fats are one of the top items on the description.

In today's newspapers and magazines you find a lot of talk about cutting down on fat. About low fat diets, about low fat everything.

Fat is an essential to our diets. Fat carries fat-soluble vitamins including E and D and A, that are absorbed into your bloodstream. Some of the fat turns into fatty acids you need to rebuild the intestinal walls that are constantly being worn away by digestion.

The problem is in the Western world we simply eat too much fat.

More Fat, More Problems

When we get too much fat in our diet it causes trouble.

☐ Cholesterol is one of them. You know about too much cholesterol, it clogs up your arteries and can cause big heart problems.

- Saturated fats are trouble. We get a lot of saturated fat from milk products. The saturated fats are turned into fatty molecules that increase blood cholesterol levels and also cause a lot of heart and circulation problems.
- Colon Cancer. One of the major problems with too much fat in your diet is that it is a big contributor to colon cancer. Your liver secretes bile into your small intestine to help digestion. Bile is a carcinogen but usually it does its work and is flushed through your gut before it can build up and do any harm.

A high fat diet increases the amount of bile produced and the result is it can build up in your colon. High levels of bile in the colon is a natural breeding ground for cancer.

Some of that same over-production of bile can back up into your pancreas. Some experts think that the bile there is one reason for pancreatic cancer.

Then when you get too much fat in your system, more than can be burned off during normal activities, it is stored in the body as cellular fat and that's when the pounds begin to mount up.

Some Good Ones

There are some fats that are not as bad for you as the others. Olive oil is a good way to go for cooking instead of margarine or Crisco. Eat lots of fish. Fish oils seem to have a lot of beneficial effects, even though we aren't quite sure why they do.

If you want to get away from fatty pork and beef, take a longer look at poultry. Both chicken and turkey are low in fat. You can cook both with the skin on, but pull the skin off before you eat it to cut down on the fat level even farther.

SOLUTION #6: ANTACIDS—QUIT USING THEM

We know, we know. In a previous chapter we said that you could take antacids if nothing else seemed to help. You can, but it would be better if you didn't.

Remember our old medical friend the placebo? A sugar pill given to some patients who demand medication even though there is nothing that any pill can do for them. Most of the patients who take placebos will tell you what a wonderful cure they have found. It's supposed to work that way. If a patient thinks the medicine is helping, he or she is often helped.

For many, antacids work the same way. Belly hurts, or gas or whatever and take an antacid and feel better. You probably would feel just as good in the same amount of time if you took nothing at all.

Some of the antacids can actually make you feel worse than you were and do you physical harm.

Aluminum hydroxide in antacid can reduce the amount of phosphorus in your system. Taken repeatedly, it can thin out your bones and cut down on muscle mass. Besides that, it can be constipating.

Sodium bicarbonate. If you take this with milk, it can give your system an alkaline imbalance and that can harm your kidneys and cause high blood pressure.

The popular brands of antacids that contain aluminum (Maalox, Mylanta and Gelusil) can cause real harm if over used. Aluminum has been named as a possible cause of Alzheimer's disease. We know that too much aluminum in the system can also lead to lung problems and diseases of both your bones and heart.

If you still wish there was something you could take to make you think at least that your stomach would feel better, try some aloe vera gel. Yes, the same herb that's used in hand cream and for first aid for burns. Health food experts say that aloe vera gel tastes a bit bitter, but that it will soothe your aching gut remarkably well. It's safe, can't hurt, so you might want to give it a try.

A LOT ABOUT FOOD ALLERGIES

First just what do we mean by a food allergy? Quickly, an allergy is a misdirected response by your body's defense mechanism.

Your body's front line troops usually fight this way when unwanted germs show up in your body. Your immune system opens fire on them with a division of cells that engulf the bad bacteria directly. At the same time other cells release antibodies in the form of sticky proteins that attach themselves to the bad bacteria. Then fresh troops of cells release a toxic chemical that usually kills the invader.

That's the normal sequence. When toxic bacteria is attacked by your immune system, you usually don't notice it at all. It's silent germ warfare fought deep in your body somewhere.

When that same immune system attacks some harmless pollen or a chunk of food or some unfamiliar drug...that's called an allergy. An allergy is a mistake made by the immune system. We don't know why these goofs happen. Maybe someday we will and allergies will be cured with a pill and all the allergy specialists will be out of work.

The problem comes for allergy sufferers when the last set of troops release the toxic chemicals to wipe out the invaders. With our pollen example, the cells release histamine designed to overwhelm this vicious invader. The poor little pollen sits there and is engulfed but the reaction goes on. The histamine causes redness and itching, and inflammation, your nose clogs up and your eyes get puffy and you get itchy welts. This is an easier one to treat than most. You take antihistamine shots or pills and usually the histamine problems go away.

With food allergies it can be a real crosstic-jigsaw puzzle. That's because a food allergy results in the release of not only the histamine but other chemicals as well that we call immunological. There are cases of food allergies that have such violent reactions that they can kill the victim. In one situation the throat swells quickly and strangles the person and the heart also might stop from the shock.

Other reactions to food allergies include abdominal cramps, asthma, vomiting, itching, swelling, diarrhea, rashes and headaches.

You'll know it when you have a food allergy. It will cause an itchy rash, puffy eyelids or lips, a lot of sneezing, itching of the eyes and nose. These reactions don't last very long. This means that the immune system soon realizes its mistake or is pleased with overwhelming the bad guy so easily, and closes up shop and marches home.

Allergies are highly individualistic. What provokes an attack in one person, might not in his brother or sister. There are foods that seem to affect people more than other foods. These include cow's milk, wheat products, chocolate, eggs, fin fish, nuts, and shellfish.

Somebody figured out which foods are least likely to cause an allergy in anyone. They are: rice, carrots, pears, gelatin, lamb, lettuce and apples. Why? We haven't heard anyone answer that question.

SO, HOW TO FIND THE VILLAIN?

Doctors say by taking a history. You can do the same thing by looking at your normal diet and simply eliminating one type of food at a time. Start by not using any cow's milk, not to drink, to put on cereal, in coffee, not to use whipped cream, ice cream and all the other bovine products.

A week is usually enough time to see if it has any effect on your allergy rating. If there's no change, mark that down on your dietary diary and move on to another food or food group such as eggs, wheat, etc. Work through all the most usual allergy causing foods. If you haven't hit your bad guy yet, look at the rest of your diet and pick out various foods or food groups you can test. Soon you'll find the one doing the damage.

During this test period don't eat at restaurants and avoid all processed food that might have your test food in it.

With most people, this will find the cause of the allergy. If it doesn't, there are skin tests and blood tests that are usually done by doctors who specialize in allergies.

HOW TO TREAT THE ALLERGY

The best way to treat any allergy is to avoid eating the food that caused the problem. But you love tomatoes. Tomatoes give you a stuffed up nose and watery eyes and your gut feels like all the Hitler youth divisions are marching down a highway to hell. Then don't eat tomatoes. You love tomatoes. Then eat tomatoes and put up with the allergy problems.

Antihistamines can be taken to prevent the itching and hives and hay fever symptoms produced by most of the food allergies. Prevention is the key here. The antihistamines

The highest thought is always the one containing JOY

The clearest words are those which contain TRUTH

The grandest feeling is the one you call LOVE.

I cannot tell you MY TRUTH till you stop telling me Yours

won't stop the symptoms if they have already started. If you know you'll be eating the wrong foods, take the antihistamines before you eat. Best, don't eat the foods that you're allergic to at all.

THE LACTOSE PROBLEM

If you're a black or oriental adult or a white from the Mediterranean countries, you probably suffer from lactose intolerance. This means that you can't digest the lactose sugar in milk and milk products.

Lactose intolerance doesn't show up in children, since nature intended children to drink milk. Man is the only animal where the adult of the species drinks or eats mother's milk products. Strange, isn't it?

If you can't tolerate lactose, you react to milk, ice cream, cream and other high milk content foods. You can eat cheese and yogurt, however, with no bad effects because these are products which are fermented and that digests much of the lactose.

The way to solve the lactose problem is to avoid those foods and milk, or to treat your milk with Lactaid to help in the digestion process. Take a look in a large supermarket and you probably can find Lactaid milk. It usually costs a third more than regular milk. Often it is available in skim milk and a special CalciMilk that is low-fat and lactose-reduced, with added calcium.

One strange contradiction here. There are some lactose sensitive people who can drink hot chocolate made with regular milk and suffer no harmful effects. Somehow the chocolate in the milk neutralizes the harmful effects of the lactose and the body can digest it just fine.

Remember, this works only for some of you who are lactose intolerant. If it works for you, fine.

WHEAT AND GRAIN PROBLEMS

Some people have a hard time digesting wheat, barley, rye, oats and a few other grains. The experts aren't sure if this is a food intolerance or a real allergy. Those few who are allergic to wheat can usually be spotted in allergy tests. But if the problem is the gluten found in the grains produces a sensitivity and not an allergy, it won't show up on a test. That makes it much harder to discover and to deal with.

Gluten sensitivity can show up in symptoms that look exactly like those of I.B.S. If you have some symptoms that you can't figure out, and they don't seem to be related to any of the I.B.S. problems, about the only thing you can do is to stop eating the gluten foods such as oats and wheat and all the wheat products. This includes breads, cakes, cookies, oatmeal, barley soup, anything that includes the grain or flour of those grains.

It will be tough, and take some figuring, but you'll find enough other things to eat for your week-long test. If, at the end of the week, these grungy little pains and problems have vanished, you may have found your culprit.

So if wheat gluten is your problem, there are a lot of foods you can use instead. The Orientals live on rice flour bread and cakes. There is buckwheat, millet, soybean, chickpea and even potato flour. Check your local health food store for other gluten-free products. You'll find a lot of them.

THE FIBER STORY

We've talked about fiber before and the importance of it in your diet and especially in creating bulk for your system. Did you know that medically fiber was considered something to avoid up until 1976? It was indigestible; how could it help you any?

Then the turnabout and now we have the term "dietary fiber." This is talking about the insoluble fibers and that they soak up water in your digestive tract. The one you probably know best is wheat bran that lots of people use, sprinkling it on their other foods so they can get their thirty grams of fiber a day.

These fibers don't dissolve in your intestine, and when the mass reaches your colon the enzymes there can't do much about breaking them down either.

What remains is a big push broom to escort all of the

wastes in your colon out the door. Insoluble fiber becomes a type of natural laxative. That means that you'll have larger, softer and heavier stools, and that the matter in your colon will not tarry around for as long as it might otherwise.

This can have another benefit. The quicker your waste products and the left over bad guys like carcinogens and your own bile acids are pushed out of the colon, the less time those bacteria and germs and gunk have to set you up for a bout with cancer.

WHERE DO WE GET FIBER?

Wheat and other grains provide us the best bet for those insoluble fibers. The other kind of fiber, the soluble kind that is dissolved in your intestine and is also good for you, comes from fresh fruit and vegetables. They also are in dried peas, beans and lentils, barley and oats. You may never have heard of them but the psyllium seeds are also a good source of soluble fiber. This seed is the main ingredient in the over the counter fiber helper called Metamucil.

The best way to figure out how much fiber you eat in a day is to check how much you ate yesterday. Check each meal and make a stab at the total. Maybe ten or fifteen grams? Make it a point to eat more fresh fruit, more wheat products, buy yourself a jar of wheat bran at the grocery store and use a teaspoon a day sprinkled on your other food.

Remember, for each teaspoon of bran, you must drink

AN EXTRA EIGHT OUNCE glass of water. That's in addition to your usual eight glasses of water a day.

Yes, fiber can cause gas and bloating and flatulence. If you increase your fiber gradually, and drink lots of water, your gas and flatulence problems should taper off and be gone after two or three weeks. It will be worth it to get more fiber in your diet.

For a chart showing the amount of fiber in various foods, check the chart in the chapter on constipation.

IRRITANT FOODS

So far we've touched on some of the irritant foods that some people find intolerable. Often these are foods that affect certain areas of a person's life. In the following pages we're going to show you lists of foods that generally upset and irritate people who have certain conditions.

These irritant foods can be a guideline to helping you to determine which foods upset your system one way or another. Test them out and see if these foods do irritate your bowels. If they do, mark them down on your not-to-buy list. If they don't bother you, they can still find a home in your cupboard.

The best way for a person to work up a food irritant list is to do it yourself. Use the once or twice eating a food system to check on its potential for you.

Look for the particular I.B.S. problem you have, or

other gastrointestinal tract upset, and work out your own list of irritant foods.

HEARTBURN

- ☐ High-fat meats
- ☐ French fried foods
- ☐ Chicken and turkey skin
- ☐ Pan fried meats
- ☐ Cream and cream sauces
- ☐ Mayonnaise
- ☐ Margarine, butter
- ☐ Wheat flour pastries
- ☐ High sugar desserts
- ☐ Regular milk
- ☐ Low-fat milk
- ☐ Other dairy products
- ☐ Chocolate
- ☐ Cocoa
- ☐ Coffee
- ☐ Decaffeinated coffee
- ☐ Soft drinks with caffeine
- ☐ Nuts, roasted, plain
- ☐ Peppermint
- ☐ Alcohol
- ☐ Chili powder
- ☐ Black pepper

☐ Citrus juices
☐ Tomato juice

INTESTINAL GAS

Irritating foods that affect some, not all people:

☐ Bananas
☐ Citrus fruits
☐ Berries
☐ Dried fruits
☐ Melons
☐ Peaches
☐ Pears
☐ Prunes
☐ Apples in all forms
☐ Asparagus
☐ Avocado
☐ Carrots
☐ Celery
☐ Onions
☐ Potatoes
☐ Radishes
☐ Sauerkraut
☐ Cucumbers
☐ Eggplants
☐ Green peppers
☐ Lettuce

- [ ] Scallions
- [ ] Shallots
- [ ] Tomatoes
- [ ] Zucchini
- [ ] Graham crackers
- [ ] Popcorn
- [ ] Corn & potato chips
- [ ] Soft drinks
- [ ] Pastries
- [ ] Wheat products

The following list cause intestinal gas in most people:

- [ ] Milk
- [ ] All milk products
- [ ] Apricots
- [ ] Dried beans, peas, lentils
- [ ] Brussels sprouts
- [ ] Cabbage
- [ ] Cauliflower
- [ ] Corn
- [ ] Grapes
- [ ] Prune juice
- [ ] Raisins
- [ ] Turnips
- [ ] Nuts
- [ ] Wheat germ
- [ ] Wine

☐   Sorbitol sweetener

So, what else can we say. Food is out there, we all have to eat. If you still have problems with food, play detective until you find out which ones bother your gastric system and simply eliminate them from your life.

For more information about food, diets, and nutrition there are hundreds of books for you to check on. Take a look in your local bookstore or your library and you'll find all that you can read.

Remember to keep it a happy search. Eating should be a happy, or at least a pleasant experience. Don't get into the habit of grousing about your bad luck with the chuckwagon. Find the foods you can eat and enjoy. Your gut is going to feel better, too.

13
DISEASES OF THE DIGESTIVE TRACT

IN THE FIRST PART OF THIS BOOK we talked to you about your gastrointestinal tract, what it is, where it is, how it works, how it can get out of whack. We looked at the problems and conditions that can arise to give you a bad time and make you feel miserable.

Those various conditions were such that most of them could be cured or moderated so you could live with them and still not go crazy.

Now we move on to the major hitters in your gut, the diseases that can erupt, do serious damage and if you're not careful, they can kill you.

How do you know if you have a disease of the bowel and it's not just another less serious condition? You can't always. That's why we told you to check out any tough symptoms you have in your gut with your doctor so he can first rule out any serious disease.

Maybe one of these times he doesn't rule it out and it is something more than just a belly ache or gas or diarrhea. That's why you go to see your doctor before you work on any home helps for your hurting conditions in your gut.

When should you go see your doctor? Whenever you want to and think you should. A lot of doctors spend half their time reassuring people that they aren't sick, or that they have a minor problem and it's going to clear up in two or three days.

This is all worth while to a doctor because sometimes he investigates one of these simple, routine conditions such as diarrhea, and it turns up something much more serious that never would have been found if the person hadn't come in for the minor problem. So, go see your doctor. That's what he's there for.

In this section we're going to be looking at the serious diseases that can affect your dietary system from top to bottom. Let's start with one that isn't tremendously serious but can cause a lot of pain and misery.

THE ULCER SITUATION

Despite what some comedians build a routine around, ulcers are no laughing matter. Early in this century there were few of them. Then they struck and soared to their peak in the mid 1940s and then started to decline. We're not sure why they happen, what really causes them, and we have no absolute cure. We do know that most of the duodenal ulcers simply go away after about fifteen years.

The cause of the duodenal ulcer could be tied somehow to the changing diet of Americans, we simply don't know.

WHAT IS A DUODENAL ULCER?

An ulcer is the inflammation and ulceration of a section of the duodenal wall and extends through the lining and into the muscles below. It's a hole, in this case in the duodenum, the first twelve inches of your small intestine. When your stomach acid hits the eruption around the inflamed area, it's like pouring alcohol on a raw cut. It hurts like crazy.

We used to say that stress was the cause of ulcers. The harried businessman with too much work, too little time, a nagging wife and three kids all haranguing him twenty-four hours a day.

Now the experts aren't so sure. They say that stress probably has some effect on ulcers, but that alone is not responsible for an otherwise healthy person getting an ulcer.

About a third of ulcer patients these days are women, and that's up from one fifth some years ago.

If your father or mother had ulcers, your chances of getting an ulcer as well is more than tripled. This much we know. But still we're not sure just why. It's also true that people with type O blood have forty percent more ulcers than the other blood types. Again, we don't know why.

HOW TO TELL IT'S AN ULCER

You probably can't tell. You'll know that your stomach hurts, or something down there hurts. It usually pains you more when your stomach is empty than when it's full.

When it hurts, go see your doctor. He'll ask you some questions to get a "history" of your medical background. Many doctors don't do a lot of tests at this point, instead give the patient a six week program of home treatment. Most patients have already tried antacids and they helped a little but didn't knock out the pain.

One common treatment is to use the fairly new H-2 blocks that stop the body from producing histamines which reduce the stomach acid and there-by reduce the pain of the ulcer.

Another treatment for the duodenal ulcer is a drug called Carafate. This pill has been around for a while. It hits the stomach and as soon as it finds acid, it turns into a thick pasty substance that soon coats the ulcer and keeps the acid away from it, reducing the pain. Proponents say this heals up the ulcer as well as antacids or blockers.

Most duodenal ulcers heal in about six weeks. The big problem with a duodenal ulcer is that once you have one, it probably will come back after it's been healed. This merry-go-round with ulcers can happen again and again for up to fifteen years before they finally go away for good.

Don't eat anything that produces more acid in your stomach. You should have that list down pat by now. Go easy on coffee and alcohol. Smoking is hard on your ulcer. Careful of using any aspirin, Tylenol or Advil type pain killers. Exercise will have no effect on your ulcer one way or the other.

If your duodenal ulcer doesn't heal after six weeks, there may be some tests in your future such as an upper GI series. If this doesn't find the problem an expensive endoscopy may be done.

THE MORE SERIOUS ONES

Even if you have a duodenal ulcer the odds are with you that it won't become a serious problem. Somewhere around 90% of them can be handled with medication and require no surgery.

Sometimes the pain gets severe due to a partial blockage of the duodenum from scar tissue. Then a patient could have bloating, nausea weight loss and vomiting. Perforation leads to tremendous pain. Now we're talking about surgery.

There are two types of ulcer surgery but don't worry about them until the faint chance happens that you need it. That ulcer that you had, we cleared up with the pills, so let's move on to the bigger, badder kind of ulcer.

GASTRIC ULCER - THE OTHER ONE

Gastric ulcers are those in the stomach, and there are just as many of them around today as forty years ago. The good news is that only one ulcer in four is the gastric type. One of the factors here as well is stomach acid. It's always a fight in your stomach between the acids trying to break down the food, and the mucous lining of your stomach which is protecting your stomach lining from the acids.

Some believe that the wrong ratio of mucous to acid can lead to the inflammation and ulceration of a spot in your stomach. No one knows for sure why stomach ulcers develop. It has been well established that people who take fifteen or more aspirins a week account for a third of all gastric ulcer patients. If you take this many aspirins for arthritis or something else, talk to your doctor and see if you can use another less stomach harming drug.

Stomach pain is the big symptom here. Again, after eating, the pain will gradually recede as the food forms a coating over the ulcerated area keeping some of the acid away from it.

Treatment for the gastric ulcer is similar to that for the duodenal kind. Drugs to slow down the acid or to cover the ulcerated section.

Most doctors worry more about a stomach ulcer than the other one. The reason is that it can be much more serious. It can bleed much more than a duodenal one and hurt much more. If your stomach ulcer doesn't respond to treatment and heal after three months, your doctor will talk to you about surgery.

The big risk here is that sometimes a gastric ulcer can be cancerous. In a surgery, the affected part of the stomach is cut out and you're stitched back together. This is no huge problem, because you can live without a stomach at all.

One good point with the gastric ulcer is that they are not prone to come back again.

THERE MAY BE HOPE

Recent research and testing programs have confirmed that at least some ulcers are the result of a bacterial infection. The culprit here is helico bacter tylori. The good news is that this bug can be treated successfully with antibiotics. This discovery could have far ranging benefits in the treating and prevention of ulcers.

No one is exactly sure yet how the bacteria enters the body. It could be ingested or inhaled, but the evidence is in and now more testing and research will tie down more and more about this bacterial cause of one type of ulcer. It's the first breakthrough in ulcer research in many years.

An ulcer, no fun at all. If you think you may have one, or have empty stomach pain from stomach acid, be sure to go see your doctor for some tests to check out just what the problem is.

14
GALLBLADDER PROBLEMS

REMEMBER YOUR GALLBLADDER? It's a pear-shaped sac with smooth walls that lays just underneath your liver and is attached to it. The liver is the production factory for a yellowish-green fluid called bile. From the liver it goes through ducts to the gallbladder which is a holding tank.

After you have eaten fatty foods, your body reacts, telling the gallbladder to contract and pump bile through more tubes and into your upper intestine to help in digesting the fat.

That's how the process works.

WHO HAS GLADBLADDER TROUBLE?

An estimated twenty percent of American women develop gallstones, the major problem for the gallbladder. Only eight percent of men have the same trouble. Of the women, whites are twice as apt to get gallstones as blacks. Native American women present an even larger risk with some 75 percent of women in many tribes developing troublesome gallstones.

Medical science isn't sure why the stones form. In this country, most of them are composed of cholesterol. A person who over eats or who suddenly goes on a low-calorie diet secretes large amounts of cholesterol into the bile. Research says that increased estrogens in a woman or a diabetic condition also mean an increased risk of gallstones.

Now, that cholesterol we talked about getting into your bile and causing those stones is not the same animal that clogs up your arteries. Different stuff somehow.

SO WHAT'S THE PROBLEM?

For millions of people, gallstones are no problem whatsoever. They begin for some reason and grow in our gallbladder and we don't even know it. Those that are too large to enter the bile duct don't try, just sit there and graze, gradually getting larger. Some small stones get passed through the bile ducts and dropped into the small intestine and are not seen nor heard from at all.

Sometimes a patient will feel some twinges and slight pain and wonder about gallstones. There's a test done that can locate gallstones. They simply don't show up on ordinary X-rays because the rays pass through the solid cholesterol like it was invisible. One way to go around this is for you to take some pills of an iodine substance. The iodine is absorbed into the blood and soon reaches your gallbladder. There the iodine will stain the gallstones.

Now when you have an X-ray the rays can't pass through the iodine in the gallstones and the film reveals the presence of any gallstones and shows their size.

Another way to spot gallstones is with ultrasound. This

is the same method used to check a pregnant woman to look at her growing fetus.

The beam of high-pitched sound shoots through the gallbladder and bounces off any hard object—the gallstones. Ultrasound is totally harmless, requires no drugs and just one visit to your doctor. The readout is immediate by sight or by an ultrasound picture. Ultrasound is also not distorted in any way by the liver or any digestive upsets. Ultrasound is more expensive than the x-ray method.

Problems arise in your gallbladder when a smallish stone starts its journey through a bile duct only to find out that there is a spot downstream that is smaller than the place where it entered the duct. Now that's a problem.

IF IT AIN'T BROKE, DON'T MESS WITH IT

Unless a doctor has been peering round your innards, you most likely won't know you have a gallstone until it causes you pain. Yes, it is a pain to remember.

If the stone has stuck in the tube in a way that the bile can still slither past and do the job in your intestine, there is no immediate problem. The trouble is that gallstone will keep on growing, it will block that bile duct and then the pain begins.

When the flow of bile is stopped you'll experience one of the most intense pains of your lifetime. You may also have vomiting, high fever and soon your skin will begin to yellow.

Your gallbladder is now swollen and inflamed. You'll be in the hospital. Infection hits the stagnant bile and you'll become feverish and get sweats and chills.

Usually lots of fluids are given and antibiotics and about eighty percent of the attacks fade away after a week. The problem is that most gallbladder attacks recur. About a quarter of patients go on to develop a perforated gallbladder or it becomes gangrenous. For this reason many doctors think it's best to remove the gallbladder by surgery to eliminate any more problems in years to come.

The way that doctors treat gallstones is changing. It used to be as soon as a patient with a gallstone attack was stabilized, the surgeon would automatically go in and remove the gallbladder and the stones causing the problem. You don't really need that gallbladder reservoir to maintain a healthy life. Without it the liver will drip, drip, drip bile into your intestine at regular intervals and get the fat processing job done.

Now there are other ways to work on the gallstone problem. The newest is to crush the stones with high frequency sound waves. For this the patient is sedated, put on a special table with the right upper abdomen under water. The water conducts the high frequency sound waves. A computer is used to pinpoint the stones, then the computer directs the shock wave to hit the stones and pulverize them. There is no pain.

The shock wave treatment is followed by a drug series to further dissolve the small pieces of stones so they can pass through the bile ducts and out of the danger area.

Another treatment method is to dissolve the stones by taking orally bile acids. They change the cholesterol in the stones so it can dissolve, but it does so at a slow rate and this isn't an answer for stones clogging bile ducts and giving you fits.

CAN YOU PREVENT GALLSTONES?

Probably not. It will help if you are seriously overweight to cut down on your weight. Fat women over sixty are the highest risk group for serious gallbladder problems.

Recent studies have shown that Mexican women now are showing more signs of gallbladder problems as well as white women and Indians.

One thing you should not do. Don't worry about gallstones. Don't ask your doctor to examine you for gallstones. If they are there and not giving you any trouble, be thankful. If they are there and one of these days they do give you big trouble, you'll know about it in seconds.

The next suggestion you've heard a lot in this book. If you have any questions about gallstones or your gallbladder, by all means have a heart to gallbladder talk with your doctor.

15
DIVERTICULOSIS—
DIVERTICULITIS

DIVERTICULOSIS. Hope you've never heard of the word. If that's true, then you've probably never been bothered by this problem of the Western World that has significant bearing on the health of your colon.

A diverticulum is a medical word for a small hernia, in this case in the colon that develops at a weak place usually near a blood vessel where it penetrates the muscular wall of the colon. Why do we get them? Prior to World War I the disease was practically unknown. It hit the medical textbooks in 1917 and started to take its toll. By the 1960s the increase continued and today over half of Americans over sixty have diverticula problems in their colons.

Why? Blame it all on a low fiber diet. As fiber intake in the Western diet went down, the incidence of diverticulosis soared.

Here's what happens:

When you eat a high fat, high sugar diet with a five to ten grams of fiber a day, your stool is small and becomes hard and difficult to move through your colon. The harder you try to make it move, the more pressure you put on the colon.

When too much pressure hits the colon, it reacts in weak areas and a small balloon of the colon breaks past the surrounding muscles and herniates. This leaves a little pocket in the side of the colon, a small empty flap.

This is not good. Digestive material can collect there and not be passed down the colon. When the material is there long enough, it gets rock hard, and that hardness and the movement and contractions of the colon can dig a hole in the side of the colon and cause all sorts of problems.

WHO GETS DIVERTICULOSIS?

It's not a disease of the young. But with our Western high fat, high sugar and low fiber diet, the young are setting themselves up for the disease later on.

Almost anyone can get this problem if the diet is low enough on fiber. Those living in third world countries and in Africa and the Orient seldom get diverticulosis because of their high fiber diets.

Symptoms are hard to come by for diverticulosis and what are there are sometimes confused with I.B.S. In fact that's how many people learn that they have diverticulosis, when they come to a doctor with some other G.I. problem and it turns out there are diverticulosis irregularities as well.

You may feel bloating, nausea, constipation, fever,

chills and sometimes cramp-like pain in your lower left abdomen. This pain can be worse after meals and when you're under stress. In these cases passing gas or a bowel movement may either make you feel better or worse.

X-rays are usually used to check your colon to see if you have diverticula and if they are inflamed.

One symptom is absolute. If you find a lot of blood in your stool or if you seem to be hemorrhaging, get to your doctor or to a hospital quickly.

What often happens here is that some of that rock hard fecal matter in the flap has been pushed hard against that nearby blood vessel and torn a hole in it, producing the blood.

In most of these cases the bleeding will stop in a few days and now and again blood transfusions are needed. This will lead to examinations to determine the damage and work up the next treatment. This can lead to surgery where the surgeon will take out that part of the colon that is damaged and sew it back together. Remember, you have a lot of colon and will never miss a little bit of it.

DIVERTICULITIS

This problem is different. Look at the end of the word, "itis." This means infection. The previous ending of the same base word was "osis" which means an abnormal or diseased condition.

Remember that bit of stool that became rock hard in one of your hernias in your colon? If it rubs the wall of the colon and wears a hole, then bacteria from your colon can get out into the tissue or even on through into the peritoneal cavity and cause all sorts of infections and problems.

Usually when this happens, your body's immune system calls out the troops and kills off the invading bacteria. During one of these battles you'll know it with pain in the lower left abdomen, but otherwise you'll come through it unwounded. Why the lower left since your colon goes up your left as well as right side?

In four out of five cases the problem is in the lower left side. The odds are four to one that yours will be.

If the battle is won by the invading bacteria, you'll get infection and a lot of pain and be really sick. Sometimes bed rest, antibiotics, stool softeners and a liquid diet will kill off the invading infection.

A lot of these patients are over 50, and the doctor will often send them to the hospital where they can be monitored better, and where they can be given intravenous antibiotics and the rest of the treatment listed above.

Recurring attacks like this one or infections that can't be whipped, mean the patient is then a good candidate for surgery. Then the offending bit of bowel is removed and stitched back together again.

HOW TO PREVENT BOTH OF THESE

If you're an adult living in America, it's probably already too late to prevent those nasty little hernias in your colon. Even if they are there, you can "mitigate the circumstances" by moving to a higher fiber diet. This makes your stool softer and with more bulk and it's easier for your colon muscles to move it through.

What this does is take a lot of the pressure off those hernias already in there, should prevent any more from developing, and might sweep out some of the rock hard matter in them as well. The high fiber diet is the key. It doesn't matter how you get it, from Metamucil, high fiber foods, or wheat bran you sprinkle on your cereal or desserts or mashed potatoes.

The whole idea is to get your fiber count up from five or six to twenty-five or thirty. Refer back to the high fiber food chart in the constipation chapter for good things to eat to build up your fiber intake. Remember, thirty should be your goal. Don't do it all at once or you might end up with a foot long block of raw fiber in your colon that will have to be cut out with a terribly sharp knife. Take it slow and easy, but get your fiber count up.

It doesn't mean you'll be eating dull foods with no appeal and no taste. Try some of the vegetarian dishes. A lot of them are delightful and tasty and they are good for you.

Oh, by the way, lifelong vegetarians seldom have any problem with diverticulosis or -itis. They planned it that way.

SOME DIET SUGGESTIONS

After a bout with diverticulitis you probably should try a soft-fiber diet. Don't attempt whole grains or raw vegetables. Steamed or boiled root vegetables or vegetable soups are good. These can be made and then put through the blender.

Watermelon, cantaloupe, peeled pears, white rice, tofu, and soaked prunes will be good for you.

Drink? Try carrot juice or tea made from slippery elm, comfrey and mullein. To help your colon fight off residual harmful bacteria try aloe vera gel.

Remember, before you have diverticulosis problems, get your fiber count up to thirty.

16
INFLAMMATORY BOWEL DISEASE

THIS GENERAL TERM, inflammatory bowel disease, is used when talking about two serious bowel problems, Crohn's disease and ulcerative colitis. In many ways they are similar, in fact some twenty-five percent of the time doctors can't tell the difference in them in early stages.

Symptoms are much the same: diarrhea, bloody stool, weight loss and fever. If you have Crohn's disease you probably will have lower abdominal cramps on the right side. If it's ulcerative colitis the cramps will be on the left. That pain and lump on the right side has more than once been misdiagnosed as appendicitis and the doctors operated only to find a perfectly healthy appendix. Be sure your doctor doesn't make this tricky mistake.

The situation of a high fat, high sugar diet jumps up again here. The fact is that both Crohn's disease and ulcerative colitis are both practically unknown in less developed societies where people eat a great deal of fiber in their diets. High fat, high sugar, low fiber diet of the Western world may be partly responsible for both of these diseases.

Once you get either of the inflammatory diseases, it's too late to get on the high fiber program. In fact, then a low-fiber, almost zero-fiber, diet maybe prescribed.

So if you don't have either of these two problems now, get on that high-fiber diet. Twenty-five to thirty grams a day, and just maybe you can avoid the pain, suffering and heartbreak of the inflammatory problems.

ULCERATIVE COLITIS

First let's look at ulcerative colitis. This is an inflammation of the colon and rectum that after a time will cause ulcers in the lining of the colon. After the disease has established itself, it will be with you for the rest of your life.

No one really understands what causes this or Crohn's disease. We do know that it's a mark of high stress and high pressure, and that it has rapidly increased over the past fifty years. Both the infectious bowel diseases have a Jewish slant. Both are from three to six times as frequent in Jews as in non-Jews. Whites also suffer these two more than other races, but blacks are beginning to catch up. Both women and men suffer here about the same.

Some experts still say that these ailments are the result of stress, environmental pollutants, heredity, food additives, poor nutrition and a generally adverse life-style. But that's a guess.

One new theory is that the diseases are caused by microbes. The evidence so far is sketchy, but if microbes are to blame, the medical community will be overjoyed. It's much easier to deal with a disease when you know what causes it.

Another theory is that they are the result of some autoimmune problem. In instances like this the immune system turns on the body and attacks a perfectly healthy part or organ. Rheumatoid arthritis where the immune system attacks your joints is an example. These are tough problems to fight.

With ulcerative colitis, the inflammation attacks only the lining of the colon, and not the thicker muscular wall just underneath. For this reason, it's somewhat easier to treat.

It is especially prone to affect the rectum area and the left side of the colon. In some patients, it can involve the whole colon. If you have ulcerative colitis, you may also develop other problems including arthritis of the spine and joints, liver disease and bile tract problems.

CROHN'S DISEASE

Most people who get Crohn's disease have attacks in the last portion of the intestine and in the colon, however problems can develop from the mouth all the way to the anus.

Here the inflammation is involved through the entire wall of the bowel, not just the inner lining. This inflammation may cause the bowel wall to thicken, which restricts the inside of the tube so much that a blockage can occur.

Problems include fistulas, an abnormal passage between two organs, such as between loops of the small intestine. There may also be abscesses around the anus and others inside the abdomen. Other problems can spin off from the Crohn's disease including inflammation of the eyes, arthritis, skin disorders and inflammation of the spine.

While no specific cause has been found for Crohn's disease, it is known that there is a genetic weakness for developing the disease. Over forty percent of close relatives of Crohn's disease patients also develop the disease.

TREATMENT OF INFLAMMATORY BOWEL DISEASE

The first step by most doctors is to rule out all other diseases and conditions. There will be stool testing and probably a barium enema. This test makes your colon visible on the X-ray. If you've had bloody diarrhea for some time, most doctors will do or order a sigmoidoscope examination. This is done with a flexible tube inserted in your anus and allows your doctor with the help of fiber optics to view the inside of your colon and even take biopsies.

Once all of the tests are done, your doctor should know if you have ulcerative colitis or Crohn's disease. He'll use steroids, cortisone or antibiotics to reduce the inflammation. Drugs should control both diseases, but they can't cure them. Many people can go for years without any flares, but the basic tendency is still there.

Here we have a situation where a low fiber diet is best. The less that reaches the bowel in this situation the better. Foods that can be digested nearly 100% are best in treating these diseases. Sometimes an "elemental diet" of liquid nutrients is ordered so nothing gets to the colon at all.

Once the inflammation is controlled, patients are told they can eat anything that doesn't ordinarily upset their insides.

SURGERY

There is one absolute way to cure ulcerative colitis, that's to surgically remove the entire colon. If it isn't there it can't become infected and inflamed and give you grief. Taking out part of the colon doesn't help much. The disease will strike again soon in some part of it that's left.

A total colectomy is a big step, but sometimes it's the only way to stop a tremendously difficult situation and let the patients get on with their lives. The usual result is a plastic bag that is worn by the patient where the small intestine empties. Over a million Americans have had colectomies and there are support groups in most states.

CANCER

The worst complication to inflammatory bowel disease is that often it develops cancer. Some experts say that those with ulcerative colitis will develop cancer at the rate of forty-two percent after having the disease for thirty years. Others say that the figure should be about seven percent developing cancer after twenty-five years. Even the experts disagree. In either case the figures are much higher than for the general population who do not have inflammatory bowel disease.

A LOT WE DON'T KNOW

Medical science admits that we don't know a great deal about inflammatory bowel disease. If we had a germ or microbe or some definite cause, we'd soon learn how to deal with it and cure it. We don't, so if you don't know what causes it, it might be anything. Check out everything.

A doctor in New York City found that some of his patients who quit smoking developed colitis after they quit. He started a study to see if chewing nicotine gum would be of any help to his ulcerative colitis patients.

Another doctor had a patient who said his grandfather also had colitis. Back then they knew even less about it and he was told he had only six months to live. With nothing to lose, he went to a chiropractor who found some pinched nerves. He manipulated the man's spine and soon his colitis cleared up. The modern day young man tried the same thing with a chiropractor. Once his inflammation had cleared up, he also ate lots of high fiber foods and he was able to stay away from steroid medication. That's one case. We don't know if adjustments of the spine can do all that, but that's the problem: we just don't know.

17
ESOPHAGUS DISEASES

MOST PEOPLE DON'T HAVE the foggiest idea where their esophagus is. We don't mind that, we're not too good on other people's specialties. For instance some don't know much about a carburetor, or the gear ratio on a car, or how to get from a computer's hard disc to all of those little floppy things.

Actually the esophagus is that tube that connects the back of your mouth/throat to your stomach. Not a lot more than a pipeline to pass along the food and drink you need to live into your stomach where the digestive process takes place.

Usually when somebody thinks they have something wrong with their esophagus, it's really a case of heartburn. We went into heartburn in depth back in chapter five. If heartburn is really what you have, take a quick review of that section, or if you skipped it, read it carefully.

The best answer to your heartburn problems are tackled on the home front with home care, and you gets lots of good suggestions back there in chapter five.

You'll need to go back to your doctor, or visit him for the first time, when you find that your heartburn hasn't responded to any of the home care that we talked about. Usually it works. If you stick to the program you can cut way down on your heartburn.

If the home care doesn't do the job, then that's a good sign that you have something more serious than just heartburn and your doctor will take you through the evaluation.

HOME TREATMENT DOESN'T WORK?

Your doctor will talk with you, examine you but probably not do any big battery of tests. He'll make you swear on a stack of medical journals that you have followed the home care plans carefully and that they just didn't seem to work. Then he'll try some drug series.

Right now the favorite seems to be the H-2 blockers, that block histamines from working in the body. They are our old friends Tagamet and Zantac. They can literally shut off the production of acid in your stomach...which goes a long way to keeping that same acid out of your esophagus.

Another one that might also be given here is Carafate. This tablet can be dissolved in a half a cup of water. It forms a thick and acid-resisting coating. By drinking this slowly, there's a good chance that it can help to coat your esophagus and keep the acid away that way. When it gets to your stomach it can't hurt anything and will calm down any budding ulcer you may have by protecting it as well from the acids.

The whole purpose of home care and the drug treatment is to give you enough pain free time to let your inflamed esophagus heal properly. This can take up to two months.

NEXT UP TO BAT

If none of these methods relieve your problem, the chances are that you'll find yourself at a specialist, the gastroenterologist, who is the expert at diagnosing problems like these. The culprit may be a leaky lower esophagus sphincter.

To find out, the new doctor may use one or two or three tests. These aren't fun or pretty and you don't want to know all about them. One is the Berstein test that monitors the pH level in your stomach. It involves a tube running through your nose and into your stomach.

The next test is called an endoscopy. This is the flexible tube that goes down your esophagus with fiber optics and lets the doctor see exactly the condition of your esophagus and the valve at the end.

The latest technique of checking out that sphincter is called gamma scanning. For this you drink a small amount of radioactive tracer, then lie under a detector that records the passage of the liquid down your esophagus and on into your stomach. If any comes back through that trap door, the scan will show that, as well.

This is the easy way for the doctor. He sends you to radiology and they send him back a stack of films of your esophagus to examine. This one hurts the least, but of course, costs the most.

SURGERY?

If the doctors find that your little esophagus bottom valve isn't working right, you may need surgery to fix it. There are three ways to do this, and they all do about the same thing. They simply wrap part of the stomach around the esophagus to tighten the seal on the sphincter.

Yes, there is a replacement valve that's been invented to take out your old one and put in a new mechanical one. It's a ring shaped device that is implanted where the old one was. This is not a popular option simply because it doesn't work as well as it should. If it is perfected so it works right all the time, it could be a big help to this malady.

THE ESOPHAGEAL SPASM

If your esophagus starts to spasm, there's a lot of big trouble ahead. A twitching toe or knee or eye isn't much of a problem. But when the esophagus spasms it shuts down the digestive tract in a rush.

Sometimes people say that food sticks in their throat. They mean their esophagus. Usually a drink of water washes it down. Repeated cases of this food sticking worries patients.

Sometimes this stuck food can also come with chest pains. The pains are remarkably like those of a heart attack. First the doctor must rule out a heart attack before he can treat the esophagus.

This can be tricky but here are some of the ways to rule out a bad heart and know it's a spasming esophagus:

- ☐ Chest pains in men under 35 and women under 40 are seldom due to a heart problem.

- ☐ If the pain flares up immediately after swallowing, it's a sign it's the esophagus not the heart. If food seems to stick in your throat when the pain comes, that's another vote for no heart problem.

- ☐ If an antacid gives relief from the chest pain within two minutes, it's probably not your heart.

- ☐ If lying down makes your chest pain worse, it's not angina. Lying down lessens the pain of angina.

- ☐ An irritated esophagus usually has as bed fellows other upsets such as abdominal cramps, constipation and diarrhea.

After ruling out a heart condition, the next step is usually a barium swallow and X-ray. The barium will show if any other abnormalities in the esophagus could be causing the spasms.

Treatment here is a little bit of psychology and some drugs. First the patient is assured nothing is drastically wrong and he or she isn't dying. Then the patient is assured that the pain is coming from muscle cramps and not the heart or something as serious. This is usually good news and often the patient can learn to live with this since it's much less than the expected gloom and doom.

Usually a prescription is written for nitroglycerin. This helps the muscles to relax, stopping or greatly reducing the pain. The pill is dissolved under the tongue and goes to work in a few minutes. It's the same medication used for angina to relax the coronary arteries and let more blood flow where it's needed.

18
HIATUS HERNIA

SOUNDS TERRIBLE, DOESN'T IT? A hernia! But don't despair. If you must have a hernia, this is the kind to have. It's a non-event. It's a cipher in the medical world. It's a simple condition that you can have for fifty years and never know it and it will never give you one iota of trouble. No pain, no problems, no symptoms, no debilitating after effects.

What can be so benign yet have a fancy name like hiatus hernia?

Any hernia is a protrusion of tissue through an opening where it shouldn't be. Hernias can be serious, even dangerous, if they come in the wrong place. However this hernia isn't either of those things.

A hiatus hernia is when a small part of the stomach squeezes up through the opening where the esophagus comes into the stomach. Because of the position it's in, your doctor won't be able to see it or feel it. He can only see it on an X-ray.

From 1930 to 1965 or so, doctors were concerned about the hiatus hernia. It was a hernia so it must be bad. It must contribute to heartburn and esophagus troubles. It doesn't.

They thought it must have some dire consequences down the line somewhere. It doesn't.

Slowly doctors came to realize that just because this little pouch of a hernia was there, it didn't necessarily cause any problems. Someone with terrible heartburn might have no hernia there at all. On the other hand someone with a large hiatus hernia might have absolutely no trouble with heartburn.

Now we know, the hiatus hernia is totally benign. Doctors don't even look for them anymore because they are a non-player in the health and survival game.

HEY, IF IT'S NO PROBLEM....

A non-problem can sometimes become a problem. The mind has a big influence on the body. Look at all of the psychosomatic problems people have when there is nothing wrong with them physically. If a patient thinks or knows he has a hiatus hernia, he or she needs to be totally reassured that it is not the source of whatever stomach or bowel problems that person is experiencing. It simply can't be the cause of any pain or ill effects with I.B.S.

So, for now and evermore, strike the hiatus hernia off the long list of medical problems that you need to worry about. We have enough on there to be troubled about, but the hiatus hernia is not one of them.

Now, don't you feel better already?

19
WORMS & PARASITES

MANY PEOPLE ARE SQUEAMISH just thinking about earthworms. The very idea that something like that could actually live inside a human being is to them so outrageous they won't consider it.

Yet the fact is that nearly half the people in the world play host to a variety of worms that live off you as a true parasite and in some cases can make you ill.

Worms in this country?

Absolutely. If you're a middle income type person there's less chance that you will become infected. But it isn't impossible. Some upper income people even become infected— simply by eating organically grown vegetables where farm workers have worms and it passes from them into the soil from their feces and then into the vegetables, especially root crops, and then into your body. The easiest route is in vegetable salads.

So it isn't impossible. Here are some of the major players in the game:

TAPEWORMS

Some years ago a typical tapeworm victim was a Jewish mother who made gefilte fish from fresh fish. The woman usually tasted the fish during the preparation and before it was fully cooked. The common tapeworm is transmitted through raw or partly cooked fish. The Jewish mother suffered the tapeworms, but the family who ate the fully cooked gefilte fish did not.

One of the cautions to current living is to be careful of sushi and other raw fish dishes. The tapeworm could be in the fish and, if it is, the uncooked dishes could infect you. Most sushi and other raw fish dishes from established restaurants are perfectly safe. Watch out for the home made kind.

Tapeworms are common throughout the world and more common in the U.S. in the southern states. Most of us eat so well that we can support a tapeworm or two and never know it. The worms dig into the side of your small intestine and stay there. They are long and slender and simply absorb nutrients from your digestive system as the matter drifts by.

A tapeworm may live for twenty-five years and reach a length of thirty feet. Even at this size it causes few problems. A long worm or several of them might mean a minor discomfort in your stomach, but that's about all.

If you have a tapeworm you could infect others. Each adult tapeworm produces about a million eggs a day and deposits them into your digestive tract. The eggs themselves are harmless. First they must reach fresh water and be eaten by small water fleas.

When a fish eats a flea with the egg in it, the egg will hatch and the larvae will dig into the fish's muscle somewhere and wait. They are extremely patient.

If the fish is caught and not cooked well, or used for home made sushi, the larvae in the fish will take up residence in the sushi eaters small intestine and grow into a tapeworm.

THE DWARF TAPEWORM

A more widespread worm in this country is the dwarf tapeworm. It's a simpler organism that doesn't require that in-between host in its development.

This worm is most common in southern states. The eggs of the dwarf tapeworm are discharged from the body of a host. In areas where sanitation is not the best, or where small children often defecate outdoors, the problem is the worst.

Children playing in the dirt or accidentally coming in contact with the eggs can easily get them in their mouths and the cycle repeats itself.

The ingested eggs hatch and produce the dwarf tapeworm in the bowels with no other host. This makes the dwarf tapeworm harder to control. This worm is only an inch long and can also infest mice and rats who also spread around their droppings with the eggs. This further puts small children in crowded areas at high risk.

BEEF AND PORK TAPEWORMS

The only way you'll get beef or pork tapeworms is by eating meat that hasn't been cooked enough to kill the tape larvae that have hatched inside the animal and bored into its flesh. These mature creatures can be long, from ten to thirty feet, and live a long time.

To propagate themselves, these worms shed a part of their body with the eggs inside. This is passed out of the human host and picked up by the animal where the eggs hatch and burrow into the flesh.

Eggs from the beef tapeworm can't infect humans directly. First they must pass through a bovine creature. The pork eggs are not so particular. They can hatch in your intestines, burrow through the bowel wall and find a home in your muscles or brain and form cysts. These can produce fever, weakness and muscle pains. Any large brain cysts can cause the same kind of trouble a brain tumor would but this takes a massive invasion. This type of brain cyst is rare in the United States.

THE ASCARIS WORM

The ascaris is a worm that can grow to be a foot long in your bowel but most are about the size of earthworms: four or five inches long. Four or five million Americans probably have these worms, but doctors rarely see them. Over a quarter of the people of the world play host to these parasites.

These worms live about a year but during that time a female can lay two hundred thousand eggs a day which you conveniently discharge in your feces. Modern sewage systems wipe out these eggs because they must incubate in the soil for two months to become viable. After that they can live for years waiting for a host.

Ascaris worms are transmitted mostly by children who play in the dirt where the eggs lay in wait. Simply putting dirty hands in the mouth can get the eggs into the child's system. In poor nations where children play outside most of the time, most children have ascaris worms by the time they are six years old.

These eggs have a weird existence. They hatch out tiny larvae in your intestines, then they burrow through the intestine wall and enter your blood stream. This eventually carries them to your lungs. They rest and develop there for ten or more days, then they burrow through the blood vessel walls and into the lungs.

They work their way up the bronchial tubes to your throat where they are swallowed. This returns them to the small intestine in a much more developed form than they left it. There they live out the rest of their lives chomping away at the food you thought was going to power your body.

Usually a person with Ascaris worms won't know it. They usually find out only if one or more of the worms is seen in a bowl movement. Then it's panic time to call the doctor.

If enough of the adult worms make it back to the intestine, they could eat so much of your food that you would become malnourished. Now and then one of the smaller worms will crawl into a bile duct or your pancreas or your appendix. All of these mean big trouble and usually require surgery.

OTHER PARASITES

Parasites of many types can cause you problems, and doctors with nothing else to go on can often mistake an infestation for something else. They think colitis, Crohn's disease, gallbladder or pancreatic problem, irritable bowel syndrome and even ulcers.

How do we get parasites inside us? Watch out for home made raw fish dishes such as sushi or sashimi. As we said before most restaurants that serve these dishes do so with extreme care and are almost always safe. Home cooking here is different.

Raw fish can have several parasites including nematodes, roundworms and flukes such as trematode. The solution to this is not to eat raw fish, or be ultimately careful who prepares it and where it's served.

Another big parasite is Giardia lamblia. This is a microscopic parasite that lives in the intestines of wild animals without causing them any pain. Beavers are one of the animals infected. Since beavers use our waterways, they also can pollute some of our watersheds and drinking water.

A single beaver defecating can spew out a billion, that's billion with a B, Giardia protozoa's every day. They form a cyst around themselves for protection. If this waste goes into a lake or steam it can quickly contaminate a city's water supply.

These cysts can remain viable for up to two months searching for a new host. If a city's water supply from a wilderness area is treated only with the normal level of chlorine, it often will not kill all of the Giardia cysts in a water. Where there is danger of Giardia contamination, the chlorine treatment level should be increased until all samples show pure.

Infestations can happen. The Giardia parasites infected the whole town of Aspen, Colorado back in 1966, hit northeastern Pennsylvania in 1984 and Mausolea, Montana in 1986.

The parasites can also pass from man to man through poor kitchen cleanliness, contaminated food, careless diaper-changing and even sexual contact.

In many areas where aliens and low income farm workers get jobs in restaurants and cafes, the parasites are transmitted from the workers into the food being served.

Symptoms include diarrhea and abdominal pains. Or it can show up with symptoms that include fatigue, malaise, gas and bloating. If it isn't caught quickly, Giardia can also mean your intestines won't be able to absorb your food as well as they should and you may lose weight. It also could mean the stomach and intestine enzyme secretion may not be in the right quantity and you could develop a lactose intolerance.

TREATMENTS

Worms and parasites all react well to treatment with different drugs. The reactions are usually quick and ends the infestation. The biggest problem here is that usually the patients simply don't know that they have worms or parasites. Since most of these worm infestations result in no symptoms, it makes it doubly hard to diagnose them.

If you think you have any kind of worms, talk to your doctor. He'll want you to bring in a stool sample that can be evaluated by a laboratory. That way, even by finding worm eggs, they can determine what kind of worms you have and that will dictate the type of treatment.

Oh, one suggestion. If you have a lot of contact with a lot of people, be sure to wash your hands frequently. Worm eggs can be passed from one hand to another. Play it safe.

20
MALABSORPTION

MALABSORPTION MEANS that the nutrients that have been digested and broken down in the small intestine can't be absorbed by the walls of the intestine and enter the blood where they nourish the body.

In many of the conditions and diseases that we've talked about before, there is some minor problem with malabsorption. We talked about them as we went along. What we are dealing with now is a disease unto itself where the small intestine becomes so damaged that it no longer can absorb enough nourishment to maintain the body, the victim starts to lose weight and, if the problem is not solved, the patient can starve to death while eating three square meals a day.

Extreme malabsorption is also called celiac sprue and it can be a deadly disease when it isn't treated. If it is caught and treated it becomes only a minor inconvenience. What happens is that the villi, those millions of small thread like hairs lining the walls of your small intestine are destroyed so they can't absorb any of the nutrients.

When enough of the villi are gone, the body simply can't absorb enough energy to keep itself functioning. There are all levels of this disease and because of that it is exceedingly hard to diagnose.

So there you are, eating more than you ever have in your life and you keep losing weight, you have diarrhea and you have no energy.

Yes, to some extent malabsorption is present in all of the stomach disorders that we've talked about. But that is not because the villi have been destroyed. It has other causes in those conditions such as excess enzyme production.

In sprue a protein, gluten, literally destroys the surface of the small intestine, cutting down all of those forests of villi. Gluten comes from wheat, oats, barley and rye grains, and so is present in bread and oatmeal and breakfast cereal and all those foods that contain wheat flour and the other grains.

An estimated one person in fourteen thousand has sprue. There is some hereditary tie that results in one of fifty of a sprue patient's close relatives also having sprue. We don't understand why this is true.

Sprue is a disease of northern European stock and their ancestors. It is uncommon among blacks, Jews and people from the Mediterranean area or their ancestors. Women get sprue twice as often as men. Another quirk of this disease: people with O type blood get sprue more often than those with type A.

SYMPTOMS

More than ninety percent of patients with sprue will have diarrhea. Often fat can be seen in or around the stool, even floating in the toilet. Long term sprue can mean that a child doesn't grow properly and will be shorter and thinner than contemporaries.

Weight loss is a sign of sprue, especially in someone who has contracted it recently.

Gas and bloating are signs of sprue, but they also are symptoms of many other bowel disorders.

GO SEE YOUR DOCTOR

If you're run down, have a fatty stool, have lost weight and have diarrhea that won't stop and gas and bloating, you should see your doctor and tell him what's been happening.

First he'll look for the common problems, and eliminate other serious diseases. Since sprue is so uncommon, he won't even think of it right away.

One thing he might check for is to see if you have the parasite Giardia, since the symptoms here do a lot of overlapping with sprue.

You'll get an examination, maybe a blood test and stool examination for parasites and Lomotril. There are some other tests your doctor might do and if he suspects sprue he'll want to find out if you have anemia, low iron and maybe a serious folic acid deficiency.

If sprue is suspected, you'll probably be sent to a gastroenterologist who will snip a small sample of your small intestine for examination.

A DIETARY TREATMENT

When the researchers discovered that gluten damaged the small intestine of people with sprue, the groundwork was laid for treatment. Now the best treatment is to eliminate gluten from the patient's diet. Do away with all of those grains and flour from wheat and other gluten products.

Corn and rice have no gluten so they can take the place for some of the other grains in your diet. Rice flour is common in the Orient, and other grains you can eat include buckwheat, millet, soybean, chickpea and potato flour. To help you here there are many gluten free cookbooks on the market and gluten free food products that are mostly available through health food stores.

Converting a patient to a gluten free diet usually will mean a remarkable recovery from all of the symptoms of sprue and should mean the start of regaining lost weight and a pickup in energy since now the body can absorb nutrients in the intestine the way it should.

It may take months for your forest of villi to repair themselves once you're off gluten. Since you'll still be run down, be sure to take a good course of vitamins and minerals.

21
HEMORRHOIDS

ALMOST EVERY ADULT IN THE WORLD has hemorrhoids. The good part is that most of them are small and don't cause any trouble. A hemorrhoid is a dilated, stretched out vein in the rectum, that foot long tube between the end of the colon and the anus.

Hemorrhoids are the result of unnatural pressure around the anus which can be from chronic constipation and the resulting straining to defecate. This process may take several years to develop to the point you'll notice it. Pregnancy and obesity are two other causes of hemorrhoids.

One medical expert has said that these swollen veins are one of the prices we pay for standing upright. If we were still walking on all fours, there would not be near the strain on that area of the body.

THERE CAN BE PROBLEMS

Most small hemorrhoids co-exist with their host quietly, not causing any pain or any problems. When trouble comes it usually means that the hemorrhoids have enlarged and are now either bleeding, have blood clots or are protruding.

BLEEDING

When the pressure mounts too high, the thin walls of the blood vessel, the vein, give way. You'll probably notice it the first time on a bloody stain on your toilet paper, or a drip or two of blood into the bowl.

This blood usually is harmless, but rule one is never to assume that bleeding from any part of the digestive tract is benign. You don't want to be that one in a hundred who has a serious, even life threatening problem and ignore it until it's too late.

Let your doctor tell you that it's simply a small bleeding hemorrhoid and that it will clear up in a day or two. Your doctor may suggest a stool softener to help protect the injured vein. Hemorrhoid creams won't do any harm and may help reduce any pain. The best plan is to move to a higher fiber diet than you now have to keep the stool soft and cut down on any further bursting of veins in that area.

PROTRUDING HEMORRHOIDS

Sometimes the increased pressure will balloon the vein to such a degree that it protrudes from the anus. This is no great problem. Often these large hemorrhoids will protrude during a bowel movement.

Lots of times they then will slip back inside. The ones that are so large they won't go back in themselves usually can be pushed back inside with a finger. No harm done here. These protrusions are not painful, but they can be a nuisance and uncomfortable.

If these hemorrhoids get too big so they interfere with your normal bowel movements, or cause some leakage from your anus and itching and irritation generally, they should be removed. We'll talk about how to do that in the treatment section.

HEMORRHOIDS THAT HURT

If a blood clot forms in a hemorrhoid, it will hurt. Nobody knows why these clots form, but there is a sudden pain that will get your attention. Since we don't know why these clots form, we don't know how to prevent them. The best preventive is simply age. Almost no one gets clots in a hemorrhoid after the age of fifty.

A clot in a vein dams up the flow and blood piles up behind the dam. This causes the vein to balloon even more and soon a lump shows somewhere in the soft tissue around the anus. The pressure causes pain and the hurt is for real.

A sudden project for surgery? No. As soon as that blood clot formed, the natural elements in the blood begin chewing away at it. Most clots like this last only three or four hours. If the same clot appeared in a vein in your brain you'd be dead long before it could be cleared. In a hemorrhoid, the four hours only mean some real-time pain.

Treating this one can help with the pain as the clot dissolves. An ice pack is an old standby. After a few hours of the ice pack, sit in a hot bath.

If the pain is too severe, you can go see your doctor for some in-office surgery. All he does is slice open the vein and remove the clot. First he uses a micro-thin needle to inject a local anesthesia. then he cuts only the skin of the vein. You may not even feel it.

The relief from the pain is almost immediate. The blockage is gone, he seals up the vein, puts on a dressing and you come back the next day for a checkup.

Before you go to your doctor, ask him if he will lance the hemorrhoid. Some doctors do but some don't. If he won't, get a referral to someone who will.

LONG TERM RELIEF

The best way to take care of a serious hemorrhoid problem is simply to remove them. If the troublesome veins aren't there, they can't cause you any pain or any problems.

Talk with your doctor about your condition. Often a patient will think he or she has a serious hemorrhoid condition when it isn't that serious.

If some kind of surgery is required, talk with your doctor about the best way to do it. There used to be only one way, cutting off the offending loop of vein and tying it back together. This used to require hospital time. Now it is often done in the office, but still means two to four days of bed rest to get things straightened out.

There are a number of other techniques in use today to get rid of hemorrhoids. Some doctors do all, some one or two and some don't use any of them. Talk with your doctor about them. They include:

THE RUBBER BAND

Thought by many to be the most common method used today for eliminating hemorrhoids, it really uses a rubber band. The doctor will use an anoscope to find the offending hemorrhoid, circle the ballooned section and snap a small rubber band around the loop of the hemorrhoid. This stops the blood supply and within a week the vein tissue dies. That part of the vein sloughs off and is passed with the stool along with the rubber band. Some heavy bleeding can occur here but it isn't typical. About a third of patients experience a "fair amount" of pain in this procedure.

CRYOSURGERY

Now on the downswing, cryosurgery works but is on the end of a twenty year run. Freezing destroys the hemorrhoid. It is fairly simple to do; the equipment needed is not as expensive as a laser. It creates little pain, but the dead tissue doesn't leave without a fight.

The result is a smelly rectal discharge for up to six weeks after the surgery. Cryosurgery here is much less popular than it was twenty years ago.

INJECTION

This method of dealing with hemorrhoids has been used since the early 1900s and still the most popular method in Europe. Here the doctor injects an irritating chemical at the base of the hemorrhoid. The chemical cases the swelling to go down and to kill off the section of the vein and it sloughs off. This is the usual method for older patients with a lower threshold of pain. It is a gentler procedure than rubber banding.

LASER SURGERY

A laser beam is like a blowtorch, it burns anything it hits. The laser is pinpointed at the hemorrhoid, often computer aimed, burns off the offending tissue and is removed. It's a quick procedure and relatively painless. It is also more expensive and not available at a lot of doctor's offices. The laser machine to do the job at one time cost $30,000.

INFRARED SURGERY

This is much like the laser surgery but it burns off the tissue with a beam of infrared light. Infrared light is invisible to the human eye and produces heat when it is concentrated into a beam and aimed at a specific area. This procedure is best for smaller, bleeding hemorrhoids. It's usually not strong enough to burn away the larger ones that have collapsed. Since heat is involved here, there is considerable pain for the patient.

22
APPENDICITIS

☐ Did you know that your appendix can be up to ten inches long?

True. But the smallest size is about an inch long and the average is three inches.

☐ Did you know that appendicitis is only half as common today as it was forty years ago?

True. No, we don't know why.

☐ Did you know that appendicitis is almost unknown in some primitive African tribes, and low in all poor countries? True.*

☐ Did you know that the appendix is a highly useful extension of the right colon in many birds and animals?

True. Only in the apes and in man has it withered away and may be of no use what-so-ever.

WHAT IS YOUR APPENDIX?

It's a hollow tube attached to the right side of the colon that probably has no benefit for mankind today. It rests there quietly causing no problems for eighty-five to ninety percent of the population. When it does strike it's usually on people from five years old to thirty.

Why does it go bad? Not sure. But it probably is when some hardened bit of fecal matter, a fecalith, gets into the hollow appendix and clogs it. Pressure mounts and bacteria invade the appendix and it swells and becomes seriously infected.

A burst appendix is one of the few elements in the digestive system that can be fatal.

HOW DOES A BAD APPENDIX MAKE YOU FEEL?

Your experience will be something like this.

First, you'll get a pain in the middle of your abdomen, maybe around your navel. These pains often feel like they come from all over your midsection.

Second, you'll soon lose your appetite and feel sick. You may become nauseated and vomit. Loss of appetite is a big signal here. If you have the other symptoms but are hungry, it probably isn't appendicitis.

Third, a few hours after your first pain, it should move to a definite place in your right, lower abdomen. This may be due to the hypersensitive nature of the area called the peritoneum. When the infection gets to the outer wall of the appendix and touches the peritoneum, the pain will surge and you'll know that something drastically is wrong.

Fourth, you may get a fever. The fever isn't triggered by the infection. Rather a temperature thermostat in your brain does that. The infection makes it think that your body is too cool, so your brain turns up the juice and your body warms above normal and we say you have a fever. To cut down on a fever you can take aspirin or acetaminophen which signal to your brain that your temperature is fine and the brain turns down the thermostat to normal and you get rid of your fever.

By now you're hurting so much you go see your doctor and let him decide what the problem is. That's his job.

THE DOCTOR'S TASK

So you go see your doctor, tell him your pains, how it started and when you got sick and that you have no appetite and now this terrible pain in your lower right side. He nods and then starts trying to figure out for sure your problem. He has several other areas to eliminate before he jumps on the appendicitis bandwagon.

MINOR PAINS

Many people have small nagging pains and if they are in their right abdomen they panic and think at once that it's appendicitis. A minor pain can't be appendicitis because the pain there is so great you won't mistake it.

THIGH/HIP PAIN

Sometimes a patient will injure himself where the abdomen joins the thigh. This is close to the targeted appendix area, but not close enough. If you get a pain there, think back to how you must have injured yourself.

NAUSEA AND PAIN

If you have these two symptoms, you know they are associated with appendicitis. If you also have abdominal pain it could just as well be the stomach flu or some food poisoning. Give it a couple of hours to feel better.

FEVER AND ABDOMINAL PAIN

Two out of four. Think about your appetite. If you're hungry it could just as well be a virus and not appendicitis.

WOMEN TOUGHER TO DIAGNOSE

Women are more complicated physically than men in the lower abdomen. Their reproductive organs are there and sometimes they can make diagnosing appendicitis difficult.

Today women with lower right abdominal pain most often have something other than appendicitis. It might be a tubular infection, an ectopic pregnancy or an ovarian cyst. These are more often found by a gynecologist than a general practitioner or a gastroenterologist, but it's something any doctor must consider when the pains are in the "appendix" area.

RELATED PAINS

Before a doctor can diagnose appendicitis, he must consider other ailments that can cause pain in the lower right abdomen. These include gallstones, inflammation of the gallbladder and kidney infections. These usually produce pain in other areas than the lower right abdomen, but there is enough overlapping of the pain areas that they must be considered.

THE ONE TREATMENT

There is only one satisfactory treatment for an appendix that is diseased and about ready to burst: that is to cut the hollow tube out of your body.

There was a time early on when various drugs were used for those with pain "down there." When antibiotics came along, they were used in some cases where doctors weren't available like on a ship in the middle of the ocean.

Today the only realistic treatment is surgery. An appendectomy is regarded as one of the least dangerous operations in the whole of the doctor's surgery manual. The chances of an appendectomy patient dying from the operation is about the same as he or she dying from administering the anesthesia. This danger is almost non-existent and is one in many thousands of cases.

The idea thirty, even twenty, years ago was that if there's an operation being done near the appendix, that the appendix should be taken out at the same time. Doctors don't do that anymore.

There is one school of thought that says since we don't know for sure that the appendix has served out its usefulness in the grand scheme of the human anatomy, we better leave it alone as long as it isn't hurting anything.

Even today some doctors will decide that you have appendicitis and go in to clip it off only to find a perfectly healthy appendix. In this case most doctors will leave the organ in place, close up and wish you well. Doctors say this is as it should be. Doctors should tend to err on the safe side with appendix problems. If they err the other way and it bursts, there might not be time enough to repair the damage that could result. In this case, be glad your doctor was looking out for your best interests.

23
CANCER OF THE DIGESTIVE TRACT

Cancer is now the second dreaded and most terrifying word in the language, right behind AIDS, which has taken over the number one position. The diagnosis of cancer is still a death sentence for many hundreds of thousands of people in this country every year.

However we are not in a crashing, boiling cancer epidemic. The records show that overall in the U.S. the percentage of cancer deaths per 1,000 population has remained almost the same for the past fifty years.

Deaths from lung cancer, the smoking disease, are still on the rise partly because women who started smoking in the fifties and sixties are now developing lung cancer.

WHAT CAUSES CANCER?

Right now we know that there are a number of different causes of cancer. Cancer is not one disease, rather it's an umbrella name for a variety of diseases caused by different agents or conditions, that do different things to the body and that will need a variety of treatments and controls and cures.

For example viruses can cause cancer. A virus can enter a cell and implant its own gene into that cell's genes. That makes the cell multiply rapidly and continually which is cancer.

Radiation can cause cancer. Radiation damages cells in such a way that it "turns them on" and they begin to multiply without the normal controls. Again we have a malignant cancer.

We now know that some chemicals can cause reactions in genes that will start them down a cancerous trail. You may carry in your makeup a gene for bladder, cervical, lung or esophageal cancer and never have a problem as long as nothing activates them. Then you may start to smoke and suddenly one of the genes is activated by the chemicals in the smoke or tar and you have cancer.

One of the causes of liver cancer is a virulent carcinogen called aflatoxin. This carcinogen is secreted by a mold that grows on peanuts, and is a natural element in nature. Growers and the government both test our peanut crop to be sure that the aflatoxin remains at a harmless level.

WHAT ABOUT DIET AND CANCER?

Yes, diet does have a bearing, but probably not as much as many purists say. High fiber in the diet is one big help in avoiding colon cancer. It could be that the high fiber moves the waste products along faster than usual, thereby flushing out the carcinogens that might be in the waste, such as bile. This fast shuffle gives the carcinogens less time to get a foothold in the colon and helps to prevent colon cancer.

Some experts say that when you cut down on red meat in your diet you also cut down on the amount of iron you ingest. Excess iron has been said to be a possible factor in causing cancer in several of the gastrointestinal organs.

Others point out that eating fruits and vegetables, especially the cruciferous kind—cabbage, Brussels sprouts, collards, turnips and cauliflower—helps guard against colon cancer. Another study shows that eating garlic, scallions, chives and onions in your diet helps cut down on stomach cancer.

The stomach is the digestive organ most affected by diet. Interesting that in the 19th century throughout the more advanced nations of the world, stomach cancer was the most common.

This rate of stomach cancer has steadily declined since then except for two notable countries. In Japan the rate hasn't dropped and may be increasing with increased Western style food being eaten.

The surprise is that in the United States the rate of decline has spurted far ahead of any of the other developed nations. The rate of stomach cancer in Germany is three times ours and Japan's is seven times ours.

FOOD PRESERVATION A CLUE?

Electricity and large home refrigerators may have a big bearing on one cause of cancer. Most apartments and houses in Europe and the Orient are small and they also have tiny refrigerators by U.S. standards.

Shoppers in the U.S. often buy enough meat and foods to last a week, putting it in a large refrigerator or in the freezer. The food that would spoil without refrigeration. In other parts of the world, much of the food bought during one day is eaten that day so it won't spoil. There isn't room in the refrigerator to store a lot of food.

In many countries, much food is preserved by smoking, by pickling and salting, and all can be bad for your stomach and could lead to cancer. Primitive people who do not preserve foods in any way and pick and eat or kill and eat their food the same day have almost no stomach cancer.

Modern U.S. food does have preservatives in it to keep it fresh and looking and tasting good. But on record those same preservatives don't seem to lead to stomach cancer. Why else would we be leading the world in a low rate of stomach cancer?

A LOOK AT DIGESTIVE CANCERS

Let's take a look at the major cancers of the digestive tract. We'll start with the top of the system and work downhill.

ESOPHAGEAL CANCER

Not a big problem in the U.S. compared to some of the other cancers. Not quite one percent of all U.S. cancers are located in the esophagus. But it is deadly. Once detected, the average time left to live is less than a year.

This cancer is at least 95% preventable. Esophageal cancer is mainly brought on by drinking alcohol and smoking. Anyone who does both on a continuing basis is one hundred and fifty-six times as apt to get it as those who do neither.

One reason it's so deadly is that it's hard to detect. The esophagus is so adaptable that a tumor usually grows large before it shows any symptoms. Then it results in chest pains and difficulty in swallowing. X-ray tests during a barium swallow will show an esophageal cancer plainly. Once it's detected, the patient should go to an oncologist, a cancer specialist.

CANCER OF THE STOMACH

Two and a half times more people get stomach cancer as do those of the esophagus. It's eighth on the list of most common cancers in the U.S. today.

Diet and heredity both play a part in stomach cancer. As we just said, smoking, pickling and salting foods to preserve them can help lead to stomach cancer. Cancer seems to run in families whether it's breast, prostate or stomach cancer. We're not sure why. Also people with type A blood suffer more stomach cancers than the O type.

Some of the symptoms here include a gradual start of abdominal pain, a sluggish appetite, weight loss, nausea and now and then, vomiting.

A doctor can tell if it's cancer with an upper GI series. If it's positive, then comes the endoscopy and biopsies to confirm it before treatment starts.

If small stomach cancers are found, they usually can be removed and the patient cured. Usually the tumor needs to be large enough to give off symptoms, and by then the prognosis is poor. Only fifteen percent of stomach cancer patients are alive five years after their diagnosis.

BILE DUCT CANCER

This is one of the hardest cancers to diagnose. It rarely has any symptoms the patient or the doctor are aware of. The cancer strikes in one or more of the several bile ducts. A patient most often has a nagging abdominal pain.

A doctor will go through all the normal tests that can detect what problem produces a pain in that region, but there is really no way to check the bile ducts. If you suspect such a problem, the input of the bile to the system could be checked.

One other symptom is weight loss when the patient is not trying to lose weight and is not depressed. Weight loss is also a symptom in inflammatory bowel disease and gastric ulcers, but all possibilities should be checked.

Since cancer of the bile ducts is usually not detected until it is far advanced, most patients die of the disease.

GALLBLADDER CANCER

Women get gallbladder cancer four times more than men do. The only good thing here is that it is a rare disease. Most women who get it already have had trouble with gallstones. The symptoms the cancer produces are the same as for gallstones, which makes the diagnosis extremely difficult.

Usually the cancer is not detected until it is so advanced that it produces a persistent upper right abdominal pain and then a serious weight loss.

By the time a gallbladder cancer is detected, it is usually too far advanced to be cured. The experts are still not sure if the gallstones contribute to the cause or spread of the gallbladder cancer.

CANCER OF THE PANCREAS

Pancreatic cancer has tripled in the United States during the past fifty years and no one can figure out why. It ranks fourth now as the cause of cancer deaths in this country.

While smoking has no effect on stomach cancer, it does double a smoker's chances of getting pancreatic cancer. Diabetics have twice the chance to get pancreatic cancer as well. Other possible causes may be a high fat diet and the exposure of an individual to certain industrial chemicals.

Symptoms here are the same as for gallbladder cancer, a continuous abdominal pain and a weight loss without trying for it. If there is any thought that the pain and weight loss could come from pancreatic cancer, your doctor may use a CT scan. This is computerized tomography.

If the tumor is blocking a bile duct, surgery is usually called for. Since the tumor is developing so far inside the body, and there is no way to do even a cursory check, the pancreatic cancer is another one that can be terribly far advanced before it causes any pain or problem. By the time it's found, it's too late. Almost no patient with pancreatic cancer lives more than a few years after the cancer is found.

CANCER OF THE INTESTINE

Here we're talking only about cancer of the large intestine. Cancer in the small intestine is extremely rare.

This cancer is more "user friendly" than the two we just talked about. Cancer of the large intestine can be prevented, it can be found in its early stages and it can be cured.

Cancer of the large intestine is the second most common in the human body. The rate of this cancer seems to be remaining about the same.

This is an older person's problem. More than ninety percent of all those getting intestinal cancer are over the age of sixty. Heredity can play a role, but it's not dominant.

Anyone with inflammatory bowel disease is twice at risk of getting this cancer. Women who have had breast or genital tract cancer are also twice as apt to contract intestinal cancer.

Prime candidates for this cancer are those individuals with polyps in the colon. They should be checked regularly.

WHAT CAUSES COLON CANCER?

We wish we knew. It is tied up with diet somehow, but no one knows how or what or why. Primitive tribes have almost no intestinal cancer. The Japanese we talked about before who moved from Japan to Hawaii and then on to the U.S. have increased their incidence of colon cancer in direct proportion to their switch over from their native diet to a more American diet.

A high fiber, low fat diet seems to be the best way we know right now to avoid colon cancer. Animal fat is the bad guy here.

Another possible way to cut your risk of colon cancer is to speed your stool through your system. Again we're talking about high fiber in your diet. When you eat a lot of high fiber foods, it makes your stool softer and larger and helps dilute carcinogens and keeps them from hanging round the bowel walls where they could get a toehold and maybe breed a cancer. By pushing the waste out of the bowel faster the potential danger is less.

HOW TO CATCH IT EARLY

The secret to any cancer cure is to catch the malignancy early. This is possible with colon cancer where it isn't with some of the others we've talked about.

Colon cancers are slow growers. Almost all of them start from a polyp in the colon. That polyp will double in size over the course of a year and during that time it may bleed.

When caught early, colon cancers can be cured at least half the time. That's a good cure rate for cancer. If the same cancer is caught when it is small, the cure rate is over ninety percent.

How can you check for signs of trouble?

1. Watch your stool. If you find any sign of blood, go see your doctor. Remember most colon cancers bleed now and then and some bleed all the time. Watching for blood in your stool is your first line of defense.

2. If you're over fifty years old, have a stool sample checked by a laboratory once a year. If you get an annual physical, this is often a part of the exam. Don't avoid this. Do it. It could save your life.

3. There are kits in drug stores that you can use to check for blood in your stool. With some of these all you do is drop a test strip into the bowl after a bowel movement. Follow the instructions carefully. Some of these ask you to test your stool every day for a week. Do this once a year.

WHAT IF YOU FIND BLOOD?

Go from the bathroom to your phone at once and make an appointment with your doctor and tell him what you found. It might not be blood. Sometimes red matter goes into the bowel and looks like blood. Be relieved if what you thought was blood isn't. Your doctor won't mind. He'd rather you err on that side than ignoring blood that is there.

If there's no blood but an older person gets constipated often it could be a problem of a large tumor restricting the flow of the stool. Slow bleeding that isn't noticed can leave a person tired all the time.

Your doctor will listen to you and then do some tests of his own. Some of these are uncomfortable but as one patient said, "It's better to hurt a little bit now than to be dead."

If these tests prove cancer, then surgery is often used to remove the entire tumor from the colon. You've heard of chemotherapy for cancer. It doesn't work well for colon cancer. Neither does radiation treatment.

Remember the key here is to watch your stool. If you never see blood in your stool, you probably don't have to worry about colon cancer. Get that stool sample examined once a year by a laboratory, and ask your doctor about any other tests you should take if you're over fifty.

If you have a colon cancer, catch it early and cure it!

24
NON-TRADITIONAL TREATMENTS

In THIS CHAPTER we're going to take a long look at several non-traditional helps, aids and therapies that might be of some value to you in working through your I.B.S. conditions or other problems in your digestive system. If you've tried all of the regular treatments and find yourself still with some aches and pains and problems, why not take a shot at some of these ideas.

In health care there are very few absolutes. What might work great for one patient might have no effect whatsoever on the next. Which is another way of saying that every human being is unique, no two are ever alike. So no one regimen of drugs, one schedule of treatments, one ideal set of guidelines will work for everyone.

It's your body, your stomach and gallbladder, your colon and your esophagus. Take care of them all the best you possibly can. If that means checking out some non-traditional methods, why not take a closer look. None of these systems or treatments or ideas can harm you. Use common sense in their application and see what kind of results you get.

Remember, there are no absolutes in medicine, and that applies to these non-traditional therapies as well.

HOMEOPATHY HELPS

Homeopathy is an alternate healing system with treatments aimed at relieving stress and promoting health. Its fundamental principal is the law of similars and is a basic law of physics.

Homeopathy has a long history going way back to the fourth century B.C. and Hippocrates. One of his principles was: "Through the like, disease is produced, and through the application of the like, it is cured." Such an idea in principle is a foundation of much of the American Indian, the Ayuvedic and the Oriental medical practices and traditions.

What this means, is that instead of giving an ill person several different drugs, the homeopath suggests a single medicine. All of the homeopath medications are made from mineral, animal or vegetable matter. The purpose of the medicine is to stimulate your body's immune system to help the healing to start.

Actually the medicine prescribed is usually a little bit of what got you sick in the first place. Only this is a diluted and ultimately safe solution of a substance that in larger doses can and has provoked the same illness/symptoms that you now have.

Modern pharmacologists will argue that the larger the dose of a drug, the more effective it will be. Homeopaths turn this around and say the smaller the dose the stronger the effect.

The *Homeopathic Pharmacopoeia* lists more than a thousand different medicines. What about the Federal Drug Administration? Has it tested and approved of all of these drugs. No. The FDA said that the dosages are so diluted that even cyanide in a homeopathic dose would be safe for human consumption. Therefore the FDA has exempted the homeopathic medicines from its control. These medicines come in the form of tablets, drops, liquids, pills, powders, granules and ointments.

Fore more information about homeopathy, contact: The Foundation For Homeopathic Education and Research, 2124 Kittredge St., Box Q, Berkeley, CA, 94704. (510-649-0294)

There are homeopathic medications for stress-induced vomiting, diarrhea and abdominal pain. One example here is the homeopathic medicine *Arsenicum album*. This is arsenic and poisonous except in minute doses such as homeopathy prescribes.

Another homeopathic medication for IBS and stress is *nux vomica*, which translates as "vomit nut." It is said to help relieve gas, bloating, heartburn and nausea.

Do these remedies work? Check into the system and give it a try. After all, the FDA has said that none of the homeopathic medications will hurt you.

A long footnote: The modern father of homeopathy was a German doctor named Samuel Hahnermann who lived from 1755 to 1843. He became interested in quinine. He discovered that when he took quinine he developed symptoms of malaria. He determined that symptoms were the signs that your body was fighting a disease.

He deduced that if a medicine first made your symptoms worse, then it should make you better as well. By aggravating these very symptoms of a disease, you should cure the disease. This is the basis today for all homeopathic medications.

In the early 1900s, as many as fifteen percent of U.S. doctors said they were homeopaths. Dr. Charles Menninger, founder of the Menninger Clinic in Topeka, Kansas was a homeopath.

After 1910 the American Medical Association and major drug companies vigorously opposed homeopathy, and it went into a serious decline.

RELAXATION RELIEF

Stress has been named as one of the agitating factors of many of the I.B.S. symptoms. What can you do to lower stress and prevent it from further irritating your system?

We get back to psychosomatics, a word which once meant an imaginary illness that was concocted in the patient's mind. Now we know that psychosomatic problems are physically real, and that there is a lot more of a connection between the mind and the body than we realized before. Your mind can affect your health in a positive or a negative way.

This is to say that can have more control over some of those supposedly "automatic responses" of the body than you suspected.

TRY EXERCISING

One way to help reduce stress in your life is through exercise. This helps relieve the mental and physical tensions that go along with stress. Vigorous exercises, such as walking, jogging or bicycling, divert your thoughts from your problems and also help rid your body of potentially harmful products such as adrenaline that were produced during stress through the day.

A brisk walk three or four times a week is known to substantially reduce your risk of colon cancer. This may be partly because it increases your bowl motility. Whatever works.

Not only does exercise rid your body of bad elements, it also releases beneficial and calming substances called endorphins. These natural opiates help you feel great.

Yes, too much exercise can give you some unhappy symptoms such as heartburn and spasms. Learn how much exercise you need and can tolerate and don't go beyond that level until you build up your body to accept it.

BREATHING AND MEDITATION

Diaphragm breathing is the first thing your singing coach will teach you. It also applies in meditation. When you breathe, push out gently on your belly and let it seem "to fill up with air." It doesn't really but now you're breathing deep in your system in a way that can help you relax. Try to fill up the bottom of your abdomen first, then push air into your rib cage and then up into your chest.

Then exhale the same way working down from the top. Now you've got good diaphragm breathing, the basis for many meditations around the world.

Now for the meditation. You don't have to be a monk or a Buddhist. Meditation involves concentration, contemplation and mental repetition. It's easy to combine these practices with slow, deep rhythmic breathing.

The first one is simple. Start counting at the end of each long, slow, diaphragm type breath. By counting you concentrate on the numbers and wipe your mind clean of everything else. It might not be as easy as it sounds. Try until you can get up to a count of ten before you break your concentration by thinking about something else. If you break anywhere before ten, go back to Go and start over again.

When you have this down cold, try the counting again but do it just before each breath. Don't know why, but this is harder. Remember, those long, slow breaths with a white washed white mind of white on white.

Another way to relax and meditate is to try relaxing your muscles. First tense your fingers by forming them into fists. Grip tightly for seven counts, then release. Now go up your arms, tightening the muscles for seven counts, then relaxing them for twice that long.

If you work all the voluntary muscles in your body, this routine should take about twenty minutes. When finished you'll be so relaxed you may want to take a nap. In fact some people who have trouble falling asleep will use this method to defeat insomnia.

The more you relax your mind and your muscles, the better you'll feel whether it's by exercising, breathing or tensing muscle groups. Give it a try.

HYPNOTHERAPY

Some experts say your I.B.S. and several other digestive disorders are closely tied to stress. Your gastrointestinal tract may very well mirror your level of stress, and you won't even be aware of it.

Hypnotherapy, the use of hypnotism as a medical tool, is well established in the medical field for use in suppressing pain and for the treatment of some psychosomatic problems. Many experts say it can also do a lot to battle stress and the part that plays in your I.B.S.

We don't know exactly how the sleep like state of a hypnotic trance helps to relax people, to suppress their pain and to foster certain types of healing, but it does.

Hypnosis can be done by a licensed practitioner, and he or she can teach you how to hypnotize yourself. Before you plunge into something like this, go to a hypnotist, tell him what you want and find out if you are psychologically suited for hypnotherapy. Some people simply aren't, others are.

If you think it will work for you, try a few sessions with a hypnotist, then have him teach you how to use self-hypnosis. Here you will control the direction, depth and the length of your own trance. You can adjust the time so you will pass from the trance into a natural sleep and wake up in the morning.

Experts in this field say that as you put yourself into a hypnotic trance, you will guide yourself into a new state of mind which can reduce your stress and perhaps even strengthen your immune system. While in the trance you tell yourself to experience a stressful experience and then let it go, and by doing so you may be able to put it behind you.

It is well established that hypnosis can completely suppress pain. You might want to give yourself some post-hypnotic suggestions about not recognizing any pain you are having in a certain area of your body. When you wake up, the pain will be gone.

Hypnotherapy can also help you relax since it aids you in meditation and your ability to create mental images.

Hypnotherapy and self hypnosis are not entered into on a whim. They must be taken seriously, studied, and you must firmly believe in them if they are to do you any lasting good.

AROMATHERAPY

Aromatherapy is the use of essential oils as a form of health care. Essential oils are not oils. They aren't greasy and are usually as light as water and quickly evaporate. They are volatile aromatic substances which occur naturally within certain plants. They give roses, garlic and all other scented plants their distinctive odors.

How can these "odors" have any physical effect on a person who's sick, say with I.B.S.?

Part of the answer is that aromatherapy is a psychological as well as physical aid. Essential oils in diluted form are used in massage. The oils are absorbed through the tissue beneath the skin and produce a regenerative and healing effect on the body.

Who says? The people say so who use them. Part of the effect of medications is the knowledge that they will work. That's the whole principle behind the placebo effect. If part of the benefits of aromatherapy are psychological, even psychosomatic, who is to say that the results aren't helpful?

People under stress react well to aromatherapy when it is given. The patient needn't be a "believer" in aromatherapy. The massage and the effects of the essential oils seem to do a lot to reduce and relieve the syndrome of stress symptoms.

Some patients say that a massage with essential oils, carefully selected to fit the pain, will control or eliminate the pain in the back, neck or the abdomen. If it works, use it.

Stress can really mess up a digestive tract. All of us react to stress. All of us have stress to some degree. For a lot of us, at the first sign of stress our diaphragm tightens, restricting our normal breathing pattern, which causes us to feel tense and anxious. This can trigger our "fight or flight" adrenaline release into our bloodstream. The adrenaline increases our energy level and when we don't run, our muscles tend to stay tense and that can cause the whole process to be repeated. Pretty soon we're ready to blow our stack at anyone who even looks cross eyed at us.

Aromatherapy can help here when a qualified aromatherapist helps the patient to learn how to relax, how to recognize the triggers of stress, and how to use the aroma of certain essential oils to trigger these relaxation responses and keep the body on an even keel. This therapy can be self-induced with a little practice and some instruction by a qualified aromatherapist.

Part of this process is to select the right oils for the persons involved so they will be at ease with the scent and enjoy it. These aromas from the essential oils can cause chemical reactions in some glands and evoke memories that can nurture and calm our psyche.

Essential oils should always be diluted in a carrier oil before using for massage and should never be taken internally.

What are some of the oils?

For a back massage an experienced practitioner would use formulas that include sandalwood, ylang ylang, lavender and neroli, all having relaxing qualities.

HERBAL MEDICINAL HELPS

Herbs, herb remedies, herbal "magic" have all been around since the beginning of time. Early man used what he had to make his life bearable, practical. He learned that certain berries or roots or leaves were good to help make him feel better. The bark of a tree, when ground up and taken with water might stop his head hurting, or make a painful sprained foot or ankle feel better.

Over the centuries thousands of herbal remedies have been created, and a lot of them remain today. Look in any health food store and you'll find more herbs and "magic" potions and "dietary aids" as they are now called than you can imagine.

Do they work? Millions of people think so or they wouldn't be on the market for long. Herbs are like any product. Say a new breakfast cereal comes on the market with a big splash. It sits on the grocer's shelves for two or three months and doesn't sell. It soon will be pulled off and sent back to the maker. If a product doesn't sell it won't be offered for long.

When these herbal remedies and herbs remain on the shelves and in our folklore for generations, it's a sign that a great many people either think or hope that they work.

What about herbal remedies for help with I.B.S. and other digestive upsets? Here are some suggestions from people in the field who should know.

WORKING HERBS

For occasional attacks of I.B.S., the British have found that capsules of peppermint oil work well. Peppermint is a smooth muscle relaxant. In a study in the University Hospital of Wales, eighty-three percent of I.B.S. patients said their condition had improved after using the peppermint capsules. These were coated capsules so they dissolved after leaving the stomach for best results.

Peppermint tea can be used to help you expel stomach gas. Ileocaecal tonic, which contains quassia, bistort, ginger, angelica and bayberry, can be used to help stop spasms by relaxing your ileocaecal valve.

Comfrey tea can be used to soothe an ulcer. Use it only for a short time because it can become toxic. Then you might try slippery elm, an herb that will give a soothing coating for your stomach lining.

Aloe vera is another healing herb that is also good for small burns. Many cooks keep a live plant in their garden. When you break off a stem, aloe vera gel oozes out. Put this on a burn, even bad sunburn, and it takes the fire out almost at once and will aid in healing.

Chamomile tea can also soothe an ulcer and spasms and help clear up inflammation.

For hemorrhoids, there are several herbs that can be made into poultices for relief. Stoneroot is one of the effective ones. This contains tannin, a strong astringent that will pucker the skin. This one can also be taken internally.

Other helpful herbs for poultices include: witch hazel, goldenseal, plantain, Solomon's seal, white oak bark, bayberry, yellow doc, yarrow, spearmint, comfrey, chickweed, wheatgrass, horse chestnut and mullein.

Herbal help for diarrhea includes some of the clay type substances to make your stool bulkier. These include kaolin with pectin that can absorb and trap micro-organisms and toxins and expel them. Blackberry root or blackberry cordial is an astringent that tends to close your loose bowels.

Chinese prescribe an aromatic combination of cinnamon and peony to help stop diarrhea.

For a bad stomach ache, a really bad one, try bitters. This is a more traditional British drink to fight a hangover. Bitters is a herbal liquor. It's available at most large bars.

Bitters is a combination of several bitter herbs: gentian root, artichoke leaves, dandelion, yarrow flowers, angelica root, quassia, Peruvian bark and bitter orange peel. Usually fennel and anise seeds give flavor and help prevent gas.

Two drinks of bitters and mineral water may just knock out your stomachache. Why? They soothe the stomach, flush out toxins, reduce your risk of gallstones, and stimulate your appetite. They also have some antibiotic properties.

The bitter content in coffee is thought to be one reason that it helps relieve constipation in many people. We don't eat many bitter foods. Probably the most eaten one is grapefruit and some of the bitter greens: mustard, collard, kale and artichokes coming in close behind. All have digestive benefits.

If your doctor tells you that you have Giardia or some other parasite and he can't quite get rid of it all, you might try using herbs such as garlic, pumpkin seeds, black walnut extract and an active form of wormwood.

ACUPUNCTURE RELIEF

You've heard of acupuncture, the ancient Chinese art of therapy. Yes, it is reported to be able to do a lot to relieve the pain of I.B.S.

Let's take a closer look.

Acupuncture began in China over 4,000 years ago. It wasn't until the 1970s that Americans were introduced to the art. There was a lot of opposition to it from the traditional medical establishment here.

Basically American doctors look at the body as a functioning machine that can break down and needs repairing.

The Chinese medical people look at a person as an energy field. They say that a patient is a microcosm of the universe, with two major forces, yin and yang, which affect a person's balance of energy. They call this chi. When thechi is out of balance, the person becomes ill.

A Chinese doctor tries to find the reason for the imbalance. He does this by palpating and interpreting twelve different pulses and by looking at the patient's tongue.

To get the patient back in balance, the acupuncturist places needles into one of some 400 points on the body. The needles are said to move energy and adjust the imbalance.

Today many medical doctors also practice acupuncture along with some 6,000 others.

Treatments have become popular with many people because they say they work. Is it partly or totally psychosomatic? Who can tell? If it works, it works. There is little pain. The fine needles feel about like a mosquito bite. There are no side effects.

If nothing else works to stop your I.B.S. or other digestive condition pain and suffering, you can always try acupuncture.

25
COUNTING FAT GRAMS & CALORIES

COUNTING FAT GRAMS AND CALORIES is one way to help you cut down on both in our typical high fat diet. Look over this chart and you'll be amazed at how many fat grams you usually eat every day.

Food	Serving	Fat Grams	Cals
Bacon:			
Armour Star, cooked	1 slice	3	38
Oscar Mayer, cooked	1 slice	3	35
Nathan's Beef Bacon	3 slices	7	100
Beef:			
Tenderloin	3 oz.	12	208
Top round	3 oz.	8	170
Top sirloin, fried	3 oz.	19	277
Beer:			
Schlitz	12 oz.	0	145
Miller Lite	12 oz.	0	96
Bread:			
Weight Watcher's			
Cinnamon Raisin	1 slice	Trace	60
Pepperidge Farms	1 slice	3	90
Wonder, Wheat	1 slice	1	70
Light Oatmeal	1 slice	0	45

Food	Serving	Fat Grams	Cals
Pita, whole wheat, 1 pocket	1 oz.	1	80
Roman Meal	1 slice	1	68
French bread	1 slice	1	100
Butter:			
Cabot	1 tsp.	4	35
Land O'Lakes	1 tsp	4	35
Land O'Lakes Whip	1 tsp	3	25
Cake Mixes:			
Angel food	$^1/_{12}$ cake	0	150
Banana cake	$^1/_{12}$ cake	11	250
Carrot cake	$^1/_{12}$ cake	15	232
Chocolate & Chocolate frosting	$^1/_8$ cake	17	300
Date quick bread	$^1/_{12}$ loaf	2	160
Lemon cake, frosting	$^1/_8$ cake	17	300
Crumb coffeecake	$^1/_6$ cake	7	230
Candy:			
Almond Joy	1.76 oz.	14	250
Butterfinger	2.1 oz.	12	280
Hershey Bar w/Almonds	1.45 oz.	14	240
Lifesavers	1 candy	0	40
M & M Peanuts	1.7 oz.	13	250
Mr. GoodBar	1.7 oz.	19	290
Gum drops	1 oz.	0	100
Cereals: with $^1/_2$ cup 1% milk:			
Alpha Bits	1 cup	1.5	212
100 % Bran	$^1/_3$ cup	3.5	170
Apple Raisin Crisp	$^2/_3$ cup	1.5	230
Bran Flakes	1 oz.	2.5	200
Ralston Rice Chex	1 cup	1.5	194
Froot Loops	1 cup	2.5	210
Corn flakes	1 cup	1.5	210
Quaker Life	$^2/_3$ cup	3.5	200

Food	Serving	Fat Grams	Cals
Quaker 100% Natural	¼ cup	7.5	227
Cream of Wheat	1 oz.	2.5	208
Instant oatmeal	1 cup	3.5	245
Cheese:			
Blue cheese	1 oz.	8	100
Brie	1 oz.	8	95
Armour Cheddar	1 oz.	9	110
Bristol Gold Lite	1 oz.	4	70
Colby	1 oz.	9	110
Edam	1 oz.	8	100
Kraft Gouda	1 oz.	9	110
Monterey Jack	1 oz.	9	110
Swiss	1 oz.	8	110
Chicken:			
Breast quarters w/skin	1 oz.	2	42
Breast quarters skinless	1 oz.	Trace	31
Leg quarters w/skin	1 oz.	4	49
Dark meat batter dip	5.9 oz.	31	497
Dark meat, roasted	3.5 oz.	16	256
Banquet Fried Chicken	6.4 oz.	19	330
Swanson Fried Chicken	4.5 oz.	20	360
Chili:			
Chef Boyardee Chili Con Carne w/ Beans	7 oz.	20	340
Dennison's Chili w/Beans	7.5 oz.	19	300
Van Camp's Chili w/Beans	1 cup	23	352
Health Valley Vegetarian	5 oz.	3	160
Potato Chips:			
Eagle Chips	1 oz.	10	150
Kelly's Rippled	1 oz.	9	150
Lance Rippled	1 oz.	13	160
Pringle's Chips	1 oz.	13	170

Food	Serving	Fat Grams	Cals
Weight Watchers Barbecue	1 oz.	6	140
Coffee:			
Instant regular, black	6 oz.	0	4
Regular brewed, black	6 oz.	0	4
Cookies, Ready To Eat:			
Nabisco Raisin Oatmeal	1	3	70
Angel Bars	1	5	74
Lance Apple Oatmeal	1.65 oz.	7	190
Anisette Toast Jumbo	1	1	109
Chips Ahoy Choc-Walnut	1	6	100
Nutra/Balance Choc Chip	2 oz.	14	260
Lance Choc-O-Mint	1.25 oz.	10	180
Heath Valley Apple Spice	3	Trace	75
Tastykake Fudge Bar	1	8	240
Frookie Ginger Spice	1	2	45
Sunshine Lemon Coolers	2	2	60
Cottage Cheese:			
Borden 5% Dry Curd	½ cup	1	80
Knudsen 2%	4 oz.	2	100
Land O'Lakes	4 oz.	5	120
Weight Watchers 1%	½ cup	1	90
Crackers:			
Nabisco Cracked Wheat	4	4	70
Goya Butter Crackers	1	1	40
Cheese crackers w/P butter	1.4 oz.	11	210
Cheez-it	12	4	70
Dark Rye Crisp Bread	1	Trace	26
Nabisco Escort	3	4	70
Keebler Garlic Melba toast	2	Trace	25
Saltines	2	1	25
Frozen Dinners:			
Armour Classic Chick/Noodles	11 oz.	73	230

Food	Serving	Fat Grams	Cals
Armour Lite Chicken Ala King	11 oz.	7	290
Banquet Chicken Nuggets	6 oz.	16	340
Budget Gourmet Chic. Caccit.	1 pkg.	27	470
Budget Gourmet Lite Pot Roast	1 pkg.	8	210
Le Menu Beef Stroganoff	10 oz.	24	430
Le Menu Lite Glazed Chicken	10 oz.	3	230
Lean Cuisine Fillet Fish	10 oz.	5	210
Swanson Chicken Nuggets	9 oz.	23	470
Weight Watchers Baked Fish	7 oz.	4	150
Doughnuts:			
Tastykake Chocolate Dipped	1	10	181
Earth Grains Devil's Food	1	21	330
Powdered sugar minis	1	3	58
Tastykake Fudge Iced	1	21	350
Glazed donuts	1	13	235
Eggs:			
Fried with margarine	1	7	91
Hard boiled	1	5	77
Scrambled	1	7	101
Egg white only	1	0	17
One egg yolk poached	1	5	59
Egg Beaters (substitute)	1/4 cup	0	25
Scramblers (substitute)	3.5 oz.	5	105
Fish:			
Smelt	6 oz.	6	212
Red snapper	6 oz.	3	217
Microwave tuna sandwich	1	6	200
Rainbow trout broiled	3 oz.	4	129
Canned tuna in water	3 oz.	2	90
Canned tuna in oil	3 oz.	15	200
S&W canned tuna in water	3 oz.	1.5	90
Orange ruffy baked	3 oz.	1	75

Food	Serving	Fat Grams	Cals
Sea bass, broiled	3 oz.	2	105
Groton's Frozen Scrod	1 pkg.	18	320
Van Kamp's Frozen Fillets	1	10	180
Mrs. Paul's Fish Cakes	2	7	190
Microwave Fish Sandwich	1	15	280
Fruit:			
Fresh apple	1	Trace	81
Fresh grapefruit	1/2	0	40
Dry, pitted prunes	1/4 cup	1	140
Fresh orange	1	Trace	69
Fresh pear	1	1	100
Fresh pineapple	1 cup	1	90
Canned mixed fruit	1/2 cup	0	90

* Most fresh fruits have almost no grams of fat. Canned fruit has little more, but the sugar content raises the level of the calorie count.

French Toast:			
Home-made with egg, milk	1 slice	7	155
Take-out, with butter	1 slice	9	180
Aunt Jemima Cinnamon Swirls	3 oz.	4	71
Weight Watchers French Toast	2 slices	5	160
Gelatin:			
Royal Apple	1/2 cup	0	80
Jell-O Black Raspberry	1/2 cup	Trace	81
Cherry w/Nutrasweet	1/2 cup	Trace	8
Diamond Crystal Orange, sugar-free	1/2 cup	Trace	9
Gravy: (canned)			
Franco-American Beef	2 oz.	1	25
Franco-American Pork	2 oz.	3	40
Pepperidge Farm Beef	2 oz.	2.5	65
Ham:			
Armour Star Boneless	1 oz.	2	41

Food	Serving	Fat Grams	Cals
Hansel 'N Gretel Deluxe	1 oz.	1	31
Krakus Polish cooked	1 oz.	3	65
Oscar Mayer Cracked Black	1 oz.	Trace	24
Russer Lill' Salt cooked	1 oz.	1	30
Canned extra lean	1 oz.	2	41
Hamburger:			
Double patty w/bun	1 reg.	28	544
Double patty, all fixings	1 reg.	32	576
Double patty, all fixings	1 large	44	706
Single patty, w/bun	1 reg.	12	275
Single patty, bun, cheese	1 reg.	15	320
Single patty, all fixings.	1 large	48	745
Triple patty, all fixings	1 large	51	769
Hot Dogs:			
Chicken:			
Health Valley	1	8	96
Weaver	1	10	115
Turkey:			
Bil Mar Cheese Franks	1	9	109
Louis Rich	1	9	103
Mr. Turkey Franks	1	11	132
Wampler Longacre	1	31	102
Beef:			
Armour Star Jumbo	1	18	170
Hebrew National	1	15	160
Oscar Mayer Bun Lengths	1	17	186
Oscar Mayer Wieners Little	1	3	28
Ice Cream, Ice Desserts.			
Bresler's All Flavors Ice	3.5 oz.	0	120
Bresler's Ice Cream	3.5 oz.	12	230
Edy's light Almond Praline	4 oz.	5	140
Sealtest Butter Crunch	1/2 cup	9	160

Food	Serving	Fat Grams	Cals
Lady Borden Butter Pecan	1/2 cup	12	180
Haagen-Daz Chocolate	4 oz.	17	270
Weight Watchers Ice Milk	1/2 cup	4	120
Ben & Jerry's Chocolate Fudge	4 oz.	16	280
Good Humor Chocolate Malt	3 oz.	13	187
Weight Watchers Treat Bar	2.75 oz.	0	90
Breyers Coffee Ice Cream	1/2 cup	8	150
Mocha Mix Dutch Chocolate	3.5 oz.	12	210
Land O'Lakes Fruit Sherbet	4 oz.	2	130
Wyler's Fruit Punch Slush	4 oz.	0	140
Ben & Jerry's Health Bar	4 oz.	17	300
Jell-O Orange Bars	1	Trace	42
Borden Orange Sherbet	1/2 cup	1	110

Jams, Jellies:

Food	Serving	Fat Grams	Cals
Smucker's Fruit Spreads	1 tsp	0	16
Pritikin Fruit Spreads	1 tsp	0	14
White House Apple Butter	1 oz.	0	50
Bama Grape Jelly	2 tsp	0	25
Apple Jelly	3.5 oz.	0	259
Strawberry Jam	3.5 oz.	0	234
Plum Jam	3.5 oz.	0	241

No jams, jellies, fruit preserves, etc. have any grams of fat. The only difference is in the calorie content.

Luncheon Cold Cuts:

Food	Serving	Fat Grams	Cals
Armour Bologna Beef	1 oz.	8	90
Carl Buddig Pastrami	1 oz.	2	40
Hansel 'N Gretel Healthy Deli Bologna Beef & Pork	1 oz.	2	41
Oscar Mayer Bologna	1 slice	8	90
Oscar Mayer Honey Loaf	1 slice	1	35
Weight Watchers Bologna	1 slice	1	18
Hard Pork Salami	1 slice	4	41

Food	Serving	Fat Grams	Cals
Summer Sausage Thuringer	1 oz.	8	98
Margarine:			
Fleischmann's Diet	1 tbsp	6	50
Mazola Diet	1 tbsp	6	50
Parkay Diet Soft	1 tbsp	6	50
Smart Beat	1 tbsp	3	25
Regular Stick:			
Blue Bonnet	1 tbsp	11	100
Fleischmann's	1 tbsp	11	100
Land O'Lakes	1 tbsp	4	35
Mazola	1 tbsp	11	100
Parkay	1 tbsp	11	100
Soft Tub:			
Blue Bonnet	1 tbsp	11	100
Fleischmann's	1 tbsp	11	100
Land O'Lakes Tub	1 tbsp	4	35
Parkway Soft	1 tbsp	11	100
Promise	1 tbsp	10	90
Parkay Whipped	1 tbsp	7	70
Mayonnaise:			
Low Calorie:			
Best Foods Cholesterol Free	1 tbsp	5	50
Best Foods Light	1 tbsp	5	50
Kraft Free	1 tbsp	0	12
Kraft Light	1 tbsp	5	50
Smart Beat Corn Oil	1 tbsp	4	40
Regular:			
Best Foods Real	1 tbsp	11	100
Hellmann's Real	1 tbsp	11	100
Kraft Real	1 tbsp	12	100
Sandwich Spread	1 tbsp	5	60

Food	Serving	Fat Grams	Cals
Mexican Food Frozen:			
Banquet Chimichanga	9.5 oz.	21	480
Banquet Enchilada Cheese	11 oz.	9	340
El Charrito Burrito Grande	6 oz.	16	430
Enchilada Cheese Dinner	14 oz.	24	570
Corn tortillas	2	1	95
Healthy Choice Enchiladas	13 oz.	5	350
Healthy Choice Fajitas	7 oz.	4	210
Lean Cuisine Enchanadas	10 oz.	9	290
Patio Enchilada Beef Dinner	13 oz.	24	520
Patio Fiesta Dinner	12 oz.	20	460
Van De Kamp's Beef Burrito	5	9	320
Van De Kamp's Mexican Classics			
Chicken Suiza w/Rice, Beans	15 oz.	20	550
Enchilada Suiza Chicken	5.5 oz.	10	220
Weight Watchers Fajitas	7 oz.	5	210
Taco shells	1	2	50
Muffins:			
Frozen:			
Sara Lee Apple Oat Bran	1	6	190
Health Valley Banana Free	1	Trace	130
Sara Lee Blueberry	1	8	200
Sara Lee Blueberry Free	1	0	120
Pepperidge Cinnamon Swirl	1	6	190
Sara Lee Golden Corn	1	13	240
Health Valley Oat Bran	1	4	140
Muffin Box Mix:			
Arrowhead Blue Corn	1	4	110
Duncan Hines Bran, Honey	1	4	120
Duncan Hines Cran-nut	1	8	200
Duncan Hines Wild Blueberry	1	3	110

Food	Serving	Fat Grams	Cals
Milk:			
Evaporated	1/2 cup	10	170
Evaporated Skim	1/2 cup	0	100
Carnation dry milk	8 oz.	Trace	90
1% milk	1/2 cup	1.5	51
2% milk	1/2 cup	2.5	60
Buttermilk	1/2 cup	2	60
Whole Milk regular	1/2 cup	4	75
Skim Milk	1/2 cup	Trace	45
Nuts:			
Cashews, peanuts	1 oz.	12	170
Planters Mixed, Salted	1 oz.	15	170
Guy's Tasty Mix	1 oz.	7	130
Dry roasted w/peanuts	1 oz.	15	169
Planters' Almonds	1 oz.	15	170
Black Walnuts	1 oz.	17	180
English Walnut halves	1 oz.	20	190
Cashews	1 oz.	14	170
Cashews dry roasted	1 oz.	13	163
Filberts	1 oz.	19	191
Peanuts dry roasted	1 oz.	14	170
Peanut butter	2 tbsp	17	200
Pecans	1 oz.	20	190
Oils, cooking:			
Crisco	1 tbsp	14	120
Planter's Popcorn Oil	1 tbsp	13	120
Puritan	1 tbsp	14	120
Wesson Corn	1 tbsp	14	120
Smart Beat	1 tbsp	14	120
Wesson Vegetable	1 tbsp	14	120
Crisco Solid	1 tbsp	12	110
Wesson Shortening	1 tbsp	12	100

Food	Serving	Fat Grams	Cals
Oriental Foods Frozen:			
Benihana Lites Chicken	9 oz.	4	270
Birds Eye Stir Fry Veges.	1/2 cup	Trace	36
Birds Eye Chow Mein	1/2 cup	4	89
Chung King Walnut Chicken	13 oz.	5	310
Chung King Egg Rolls Shrimp	3.6 oz.	6	200
La Choy Pork Egg Roll	3 oz.	5	150
Take Out:			
Chicken teriyaki	3/4 cup	27	399
Chop suey with pork	1 cup	24	425
Pancakes and Waffles:			
From Mixes Made At Home:			
Hungry Jack Blueberry	3 4-inch	15	320
Aunt Jemima Buckwheat	3 4-inch	8	230
Hungry Jack Buttermilk	3 4-inch	11	240
Hungry Jack Packets	3 4-inch	3	180
Arrowhead Griddle Lite	1/2 cup	3	260
Estee Pancake Mix	3 3-inch	0	100
Pancakes with butter, syrup	3 4-inch	14	519

Pasta

* Most pastas are 1 gram of fat per 2 oz. The differential here is what is put in the pasta or on it. Calories for plain pasta range from 160 per 2 oz. to 210.

Food	Serving	Fat Grams	Cals
Dry pasta, all types	2 oz.	1	210
Pasta dinners, frozen:			
Banquet Entree Primavera	7 oz.	3	140
Banquet Macaroni & Cheese	7 oz.	11	260
Budget Gourmet Stroganoff	1 pkg	12	290
Budget Gourmet Cheese Manicotti	1 pkg	25	430
Dining Light Fettucini	9 oz.	12	290
Green Giant Cheese Tortellini	1 pkg	9	260
Healthy Choice Fettucini	8.5 oz.	4	240

Food	Serving	Fat Grams	Cals
Kid Cuisine Macaroni, Franks	9 oz.	15	360
Le Menu Light Tortellini	8 oz.	8	250
Lean Cuisine Rigatoni, Meat	10 oz.	10	260
Morton Macaroni & Cheese	6.5 oz.	14	290
Swanson Spaghetti Meat Balls	13 oz.	18	490
Weight Watchers Manicotti	10 oz.	8	260

Pickles: All cucumber pickles have either 0 grams of fat or a trace.

Pie:

Frozen:

Banquet Apple	1 slice	11	250
Sara Lee Apple	1 slice	12	280
Mrs. Smith's Apple Natural	1 slice	22	420
Banquet Banana	1 slice	10	180
Mrs. Smith's Blueberry	1 slice	17	380
Banquet Lemon	1 slice	9	170
Banquet Pumpkin	1 slice	8	200

Baked Ready to Eat:

Apple	1 slice	18	405
Creme	1 slice	23	455
Lemon meringue	1 slice	14	355

Pizza:

Frozen:

Celeste Deluxe	8 oz. slice	32	600
Fox Deluxe Sausage	1/2 pizza	13	260
Jeno's 4 Pack Cheese	1 pizza	8	160
Jeno's Crisp Sausage	1/2 pizza	16	300
Pappalo's French Pepperoni	1 pizza	20	410
Totino's Bacon Party	1/2 pizza	20	370
Totino's Mexican Style	1/2 pizza	21	380
Weight Watcher's Cheese	7 oz.	7	300

Popcorn:

Jiffy Pop Microwave Butter	4 cups	7	140

Food	Serving	Fat Grams	Cals
Newman's Microwave Light	3 cups	3	90
Redenbacher Gourmet Original	3 cups	4	80
Pillsbury Microwave Butter	3 cups	13	210
Ultra Slim-Fast Lite	1/2 oz.	2	60
Weight Watcher's Ready Eat	.7 oz.	3	90

Salad Dressing:
Ready To Use:

Food	Serving	Fat Grams	Cals
Catalina	1 tbsp	1	15
Diamond Crystal Blue Cheese	1 tbsp	1	20
Kraft Bacon & Tomato	1 tbsp	7	70
Kraft Free Catalina Nonfat	1 tbsp	0	20
Ott's Italian Chef	1 tbsp	9	80
Newman's Olive & Vinegar	1 tbsp	9	80
Seven Seas Free Ranch Nonfat	1 tbsp	0	16

Ready To Use Lite:

Food	Serving	Fat Grams	Cals
Estee Blue Cheese	1 tbsp	Trace	8
Herb Magic Vinaigrette	1 tbsp	0	6
Kraft French	1 tbsp	1	20
Magic Mountain Blue Cheese	1 tbsp	Trace	5
S&W Italian No Oil	1 tbsp	0	2
Ultra Slim-Fast	1 tbsp	Trace	6
Weight Watcher's Russian	1 tbsp	5	50

Sausage:

Food	Serving	Fat Grams	Cals
Oscar Mayer Bratwurst Smoked	2.7 oz.	21	237
Perdue Turkey Patties	1.3 oz.	4	61
Armour Country Sausage	1 oz.	11	110
Hebrew National Knockwurst	3 oz.	25	260
Oscar Mayer Polish	2.7 oz.	20	229
Armour Link Pork Sausage	1 oz.	11	110
Perdue Sweet Italian Turkey	2 oz.	6	94

Soda Drinks:

All but four of the popular soft drinks now on the market have no fat grams at all. Of the four that do, two are root beer, one a ginger ale and the other a wild berry. Calories vary but go from a low of a trace in diet drinks to 190. Most are about 75 or 80 calories. No big worry about fat grams from soft drinks.

Food	Serving	Fat Grams	Cals
Soup:			
Canned:			
Healthy Choice Bean & Ham	7.5 oz.	4	220
Campbell Bean w/Bacon	8 oz.	4	140
College Inn Beef Broth	7 oz.	0	16
Campbell Beef Noodle	8 oz.	3	70
Lipton Beef Noodle	8 oz.	Trace	85
Goya Black Bean	7.5 oz.	4	160
Gold's Borscht	8 oz.	0	100
Health Valley Chicken Broth	7.5 oz.	2	35
Campbell Chicken Corn Chowder	11 oz.	21	340
Pritikin Lentil	7 oz.	0	100
Snow's Clam Chowder	7.5 oz.	2	70
Health Valley Minestrone	7.5 oz.	3	130
American New England Chowder	4 oz.	6	145
Pritikin Split Pea	7.5 oz.	Trace	130
Campbell Tomato 2% milk	8 oz.	2	90
Campbell Vegetable	8 oz.	2	90
Turkey:			
Fresh:			
Louis Rich Breast	1 oz.	2	50
Perdue Breast Fillets	1 oz.	Trace	28
Louis Rich Breast Steaks	1 oz.	Trace	40
Perdue Fresh Drumsticks	1 oz.	2	36
Bill Mar Ground Turkey	3 oz.	12	163
Louis Rich Thighs	1 oz.	4	65
Shady Brook Wings	3 oz.	6	130
Whole Turkey	3.5 oz.	10	200

Food	Serving	Fat Grams	Cals
Vegetables:			
Hanover broccoli, cauliflower	1/2 cup	0	20
Broccoli, cauliflower, carrots with cheese sauce	1/2 cup	6	89
Chinese stir fry	1/2 cup	Trace	36
Japanese stir fry	1/2 cup	Trace	29
Mixed vegetables w/onion	1/3 cup	5	97
Oriental blend	1/2 cup	0	25
Peas, onions, cheese sauce	1/2 cup	6	126
Stew vegetables	3 oz.	Trace	50
Peas & onions cooked	1/2 cup	Trace	40
Fresh zucchini	1/2 oz.	Trace	3
Canned tomatoes	1/2 cup	Trace	40
Canned spinach	1/2 cup	0	25
Fresh shallots, chopped	1 tbsp	Trace	7
Sauerkraut, canned	1/2 cup	0	20
Fresh baked potato	5 oz.	Trace	220
Canned peas	1/2 cup	0	90
Canned corn	1/2 cup	0	70
Canned carrots	1/2 cup	0	20
Yogurt:			
Cabot all flavors	8 oz.	3	220
Apples 'N Spice No-fat	8 oz.	Trace	190
Black Cherry Classic	8 oz.	6	230
Colombo Blueberry Classic	8 oz.	6	230
Dannon Blueberry No-fat	8 oz.	0	100
Yoplait Blueberry Original	6 oz.	3	190
Knudsen Lemon w/Aspartame	8 oz.	0	70
La Yogurt Peach	6 oz.	4	190
Mountain High Plain	8 oz.	9	200
Meadow Gold Raspberry Sundae	8 oz.	4	250
New Country Strawberry	6 oz.	2	150